" Food For Thought " and Illustrations

By: William E. Hardison

William E. (Bill) Hardison

ABOUT THE AUTHOR AND THE BOOK

I was born and raised in Wilmington, NC, schooled and graduated from New Hanover High in 1948, and participated in various sports before and after graduation.

In 1949 I entered the U.S. Air Force and completed four years of service, stationed in Texas, Washington, D.C., Guam and Florida.

Art work was my main duty and hobby at that time.

I came to Newport News, VA in 1952 and worked for the shipyard until 1955, at which time I gained employment with the C.&O. railroad, now known as C.S.X. Corp.

I retired in 1987 after thirty-three years of service. In the 1970's, I was actively involved in coaching Little League Ball in Deer Park, Newport News, VA.

I married Barbara Duling, a Newport News native, in 1955, and we have three children and eight grandchildren. I started writing verses in 1995 with an effort to touch on the many aspects that enter our lives.

My verses are strictly of a homespun nature which I believe capture the ingredients of life that we all can identify with, so I know they will be enjoyed.

If you are indeed touched in some way by their contents, then I feel my writing has not been in vain.

W.E. Hardison

"Food for thought"
(revised renditions of "Bills Ideals" with many new additional verses included.)

ISBN 0-9658589-1-x

Published by William E. Hardison
Illustrations by William E. Hardison

Food for Thought

First printing, 1999

CONTENTS

CHAPTER I - HUMOR

CONTENTS

CHAPTER II - INSPIRATIONS

CONTENTS

CHAPTER II - INSPIRATIONS

CHAPTER III - TURMOIL

CONTENTS

CHAPTER III - TURMOIL

CHAPTER IV - IDEALS

CONTENTS

CHAPTER IV - IDEALS

CHAPTER V - MEMORIES

CONTENTS

CHAPTER V - MEMORIES

HUMOR

THE "JACK LEG" CARPENTER

I love to build and hammer nails, use level, square and saw,
but in my work it never fails, I find a constant flaw!
That in my work there seems to be a fact that brings a tear,
it turns into a mystery when pencils disappear!
I search beneath each block of wood, each tool that lies around,
I sift the sawdust really good, but pencil can't be found!
I bring to work 'bout three or four to make sure there's enough
but should have brought at least four more to make my job less tough!

But when I build I'm all athrill, my ego's miles up high,
for all those pencils that I spill I'll find them bye and bye.
And on the job there seems to lurk a trend to misplace things,
I'm so excited in my work, my pencils all take wings.
But often times when on the look the answer will come clear,
that after searching every nook, I find one on my ear!
I'm just a jack-leg carpenter I thrive on what I do...
But complications will occur when working in a stew,

but end results are always found, the best I shall attain;
although I strow things all around sometimes will bring me pain!
You know about my pencils too I always seem to lose,
but worst than those utensils few, are hammers that I use.
They are the worst of any tool that finds a place to hide.
I'm feeling like a bumbling fool when searching every side.
The hammer's so elusive when I lay it down a lot,
and problem gets abusive then when lost up there on top;

on the high rung of my ladder which I move around to tread,
and nothing is more sadder when the hammer hits my head!
It's not a way to find it there, up where the thing has lain,
especially when it parts your hair and causes all that pain.
Now you would think a guy would learn to keep it on his side;
and be a jack-leg's main concern to keep his eyes real wide,
and try to keep things organized, if he intends to build,
and do it all in safety-wise... instead of getting killed!

❖❖❖❖❖

SPELLBOUND

I didn't know at first
that driving brought a curse,
but fifty years I spent behind the wheel,
there came some in my drives
and some were no surprise,
as I saw these mysteries unveil!

Now I'll cite one on a route
that leads both north and south,
it's a bridge that lies 'anear Virginia's line,
it sits within a curve,
an overpass to swerve,
and always there to taunt my mind!

Only sixty yards at best
from each end to its crest,
but to the cars it makes no never mind,
'cause either way I came
it's always been the same.
I pass another auto every time.

It's a highway bridge, and curve,
that tests my very nerve,
and one that I shall ne'er forget,
for I can't believe my eyes
when I get up on the rise,
comes a passing car there you can bet!

But here's the strangest things
of the mystery that it brings,
there is no other curve for quite a ways.
It's straight as it can be,
no other cars to see,
and me it never ceases to amaze!

Just sixty yards of span
of two hundred miles that ran,
this incident occurs each instant time,
it could happen anywhere
along that highway there,
and not just on this bridge that's in a blind.

There are strange things on the road
that lives by their own code,
and we can only try to toe the line;
and keep our wits about
and not to figure out
the unbeknowns out there we often find.

So, I found another way
to beat the odds at bay.
I take a detour down around a mill.
It's an old sawdust road
that saw a many load,
but good enough to break this jinx and spell.

But behold and alas,
o'er this dirt road I pass,
I see the crossing bridge from afar,
as I look up to that ridge
to the center of the bridge,
You guessed it! There goes that only car!

❖❖❖❖❖

THE MARKETEERS

There's a frenzy going on that many folks are prone;
when it comes to a weekend rummage sale.
They rise on Friday morn before the light is born
and head out on the bargain trail!
They park along the curb
with intentions to disturb,
'cause they hurry up to knock upon your door;
to rouse you out of bed
so they can get ahead,
to see the things you have in store.

They will even lend a hand to give their eyes a scan,
and help you put the mess out on the lawn.
They want to have a chance to get in that first glance,
to get the best of "goodies" and be gone!
So they'll swarm around your yard,
in places where they're barred,
like your attic, and even in your house;
but when you count your take,
no money did you make,
'cause all they ever did was browse!

Next, you got up Saturday morning
while the dark was still adorning,
and all prepared to meet the rushing throng:
and breakfast tasted swell before the daylight fell,
and you're all geared up to sell,
but not one single person came along!
So, that's the way it is when you deal with marketeers,
you really have to have it or you don't;
you can hoard junk all those years,
but if no value there appears,
'Tis only fine antiques that they want.

❖❖❖❖❖

INVASION AND D-DAY

It won't be long before they're gone, these furry woodland pests;
a vicious throng who digs my lawn and makes my home their nests.
They come from every nook and cove to all my trees around;
so they can take advantage of the best of all high ground.
So, here we are, no holds to bar, we're in two different worlds,
where many spars have turned to wars between me and the squirrels.

It's here they roam, my lot and home, I'm bound to keep it sound.
The garden, lawn and fruit trees grown are targets they surround.
So, scene is set and you can bet each one will hold his own
in greatest fret the worlds seen yet; my yard is our war zone!
Now here they come in sneaky style, they creep in from the trees,
some stop to pile and dig awhile while others clip the leaves.

Some scan with glee my pecan tree and some just scratch beneath.
Their purpose is to conquer me, their weapons are their teeth!
They're robbing birds of all the seed which robs me of my plan;
to do a deed for birds to feed which squirrels don't understand.
They also flaw the limbs they knaw that clutters house and lawn.
They clip and nip and chaw and claw and it resumes at dawn.

They chew up all things in their sight, all hell is now to pay!
They dig the twigs from morn to night; my response will come today.
Which is D-Day and I must say I'm starting my offense;
I have a way to make them pay and one that makes good sense.
'Cause since a squirrel is born to sate and chewing is his trend,
and this main trait will seal his fate and one that does him in!

'Cause I concoct a simple box that opens on each end,
and on the top I set two locks and drill a hole within.
And through this hole I thread a pole where clings an ear of corn
and when the squirrel comes "in the fold" a "sucker" now is born!
When he explores what he adores the squirrel is quickly latched,
'cause he deploys those-two end doors which corn and pole attached.

A line is drawn, the squirrels are gone, they transferred miles away...
to other lands where they will spawn to come another day.
Though may it be, he'll come to see squirrel boxes all around,
and though he fancies to be free, that's bad for this "nut hound"!
So, without a gun for now I've won, I have no problem mired;
I see not one, the job is done, and not one shot was fired!

❖❖❖❖❖

THE DUEL

Man builds and toils, and tills the soils to have the greenest lawn.
To fill this need he sows the seed, then waters night 'til dawn.
He pampers it and tampers it, he thatches and he mows;
He aerates, anticipates the beauty that it grows.
But there are those who bring forth woes afield to test man's will,
Puts him on guard to rid the yard of foes that he must deal.
And they are things that nature brings which knows no boundary lines,
The dreadful sights that man now fights, the first, the dandelions!
They fill the air from everywhere and settle way down deep;
They multiply before your eye in one humongous sweep...
You kneel and crawl to dig them all, to clear the entire tract,
But all your pain has been in vain for they keep coming back!

The second one that's sure to come, most pesty of them all,
Is sneaky squirrels with tails all curled who digs in early fall.
Without regard they fill the yard with many holes and limbs,
And test your mind with what you find of everything they trimmed.
They also steal the bird's main meal...the menu is their seed...
And cost is high to meet supply for all of them to feed.
The other ones are earthly bums who burrow through the night,
And build those mounds while making rounds are ground moles-out of sight!
They raise the crown of lawn around, your hard work finds the drain,
Unless solutions can be found there'll be no grass again.
There are some tips proclaimed as pips, not always proven firm,
Is rid the ground of this worm hound by killing off the worm.

For when you spray in your dismay, it's grass you only kill,
And testy vole or messy mole still will build his hill.
Some feed this bum with chewing gum to choke him to his death,
But all it does is what he loves, is sweetens up his breath.
So they intrude in multitude, these three worst musketeers,
The squirrel in all his busy world, the weed, and mole in theirs.
Now man's awake with choice to make...and that's to choose between...
To till and toil, to muck and moil,...or paint the whole yard green!

❖❖❖❖❖

STOMPING DOWN AT BUCKROE

It happens down at Buckroe Beach along the sandy dunes,
where all and each go to beseech nostalgic big band tunes;
and many times when I arrive "I get right in the groove",
I come alive with jute box jive with every kind of "move".
So, I'm dancing down at Buckroe to old-time tunes I hear,
recalling glow from songs I know, that comes from yesteryear.

They're urging me to "bring it on" to come and "cut a rug",
and hold my own to every tone to do the "jitterbug";
to tunes they play Glenn Miller's way, to Dorsey's gold trombone,
or swing and sway with Sammy Kaye, or Randolf's saxophone.
To hear Gene Krupa on a drum, or Harry James, his horn,
my mind is numb of music from the best 'twas ever born!

They bring back memories of the "suit" called "zoot" with chains in style,
a big bow tie and wide hat high that goes way back awhile.
So all around the floor I hop, I skip, and twirl with bliss.
Although I'm "hot" I just forgot "I'm too damn old for this!"

My heart is filled with joys galore, my mind is filled with glee,
but on the floor my legs are sore, and feet are killing me!
Ah! But sounds of drums and brass trombones, of clarinets and more,
the trumpets drone, the saxophone, all heard o'er Buckroe shore.
This music goes forever more in sunshine or in rain,
for what's in store, what's one more sore! I'm coming back again!

❖❖❖❖❖

LEAVE 'EM ALONE

There is a magical splendor that seems to grip us all;
when cold winds blow, and fire lights glow; when all
the leaves will fall.
We find our glee in ecstasy, but restless in our spell,
for out we gaze into a maze of leaves that just have fell.

When leaves have died I look outside to see them on the ground,
I have to go because I know there's more that will come down.
And from my view with spirit new, I feel it's calling now.
Although the wind may not descend, I'll rake them anyhow!

So out I go to meet the flow of leaves from everywhere,
and for a while I had a pile, but now, they're ---up in air!
But never mind there's more to find, it's early in the fall;
for months it takes and many rakes-- before I get them all.

It's all for room which I assume makes way for many more,
so on I rake for just fun's sake, that raking has in store.
Yet, still they fall and sail and sprawl in showers of display,
and on and on the leaves are blown, but I'm raking anyway!!

But this is fall I meet the call, but I am not alone,
'cause from my view I see you out raking leaves that's blown.
Wow!! Still they come, it's never done, this raking, raking on,
and now it's I who wonders why that I became so prone.
I know these leaves from all the trees near other homes I've found;
come's from winds that blows and sends them all to my home
ground.

But I am bound to rake the ground although it sweats my brow--
to rake in winds, it never ends, but I'm raking anyhow!
But what if we should wait and see... just where the leaves end up,
then only then we'll know just when--- to get them
up...A-BRUPT!!!

❖❖❖❖❖

WHAT ARE THE ODDS?

Now, many people play the odds in poker, dice or races,
but there are odds we find in jobs as well as other cases.
There was a time which comes to mind, a rare, unusual case;
at work one day on our railway where fate will start its pace.

For Sam and I had worked a job the entire month of June,
and what would later be so odd, would happen very soon!
Now speak of odds, you won't believe this story here I tell;
for Sam and I would both take leave from Newport News -- a spell.

But neither of us spoke of it and neither knew each plan,
and we continued on the shift both me and my pal Sam;
and when we left the job that night we both went separate ways.
I went home to plan my flight, and Sam, to plan his days.

My destination... Florida, Clearwater and its beach,
down the west coast corridor, a thousand miles to reach!
My "side kick" Sam had no idea of my vacation time,
and I just thought that he'd appear to work back on the line.
So, I reached my destination...Clearwater, Tampa Bay,
was there a week's duration, 'til I went to see a fray,

a baseball game in old "St Pete", some fifty miles away.
The White Sox and the Yankees meet in "Grapefruit League" they play,
and when the game had ended there among 12 thousand fans,
two faces met... I do declare! 'twas mine and my friend Sam's!

❖❖❖❖❖

TOP O' THE HEAP

He's the salvage man from Denbigh,
he's the best in all the land,
and rises every morn at "crack of day."
He goes out like a dart to get an early start
to fetch the "goodies" folks have thrown away.
He's the darndest bargain hunter that ever hit the road
and has a busy nose just like a hound;
he can smell a piece of brass, or copper just as fast,
or any other "pickings" found around.

He's the salvage man from Denbigh
and the symbol of the street,
who's out there on the look come rain or sun;
he has two eagle eyes to seek out his supplies---
before the city dumpster makes it's run!
He's the best of all the like
that e're came down the pike,
with a will that humbles all the salvage men,
and always as of course there is a "driving force"
to search a trash pile--- end to end!

He's a master at this art for he knows just what to cart,
and his friends all call him "King of Rust."
He can take a 'lectric fan and make it run again,
and like it never saw a grain of dust...
or find a rusty table lamp that saw a better day,
or some old chair that's rocked it's last goodbye.
Like an artist through and through
he makes 'em all look new,
before anyone can bat an eye!

Now, he's the salvage man from Denbigh
and he does it every day,
'cause he's retired with nothing else to do,
and he has it in his blood--like a flower has it's bud;
a true trash "picker" through and through!

He’s a craftsman of a trashman
who does a lot of good,
to save those items from their destined end;
from some lasting earthly grave
back to beauty that was saved;
back in somebody's home to shine again!

So, he’s the salvage man from Denbigh,
and the richest man on earth,
and not because he handles lots of cash;
but because he feels like kings
with excitement that it brings,
and when his treasures come from people’s trash!

❖❖❖❖❖

RAGS AND RICHES

This married pair has naught to spare but try to do their best...
To make their way from day to day to meet life's grueling test.
He loves to roam away from home just like a maverick,
But she is sound in ways she's found to make their marriage click.
They are a pair with average care and usually make with less;
But he has dreams for wealth it seems, well my tale here tells the rest.
So here's the way he spent his day, and you can surely bet:
That it's to be a winning spree, - never been equaled yet!

He felt forlorn this early morn while searching for relief;
His lovely wife who filled his life came on to spare his grief.
She knew his vice, it should suffice to calm her husband's ills,
So with a wish she gave a kiss, and two one dollar bills.
So off he went with mind set bent to find his favorite game,
To meet his vice in rolling dice without a guilt of shame.
It came real soon, he heard its tune as dice spun off a board.
He joined that clan and warned each man, "no cheatin' is deplored!"

So he grabbed those dice like cats do mice, and laid two dollars down;
And in short while he won a pile and cleaned out all around.
Now off he drove to "Coco Grove", a bar with back room parlors;
His cash has come to one big sum, to total three hundred dollars.
First he sets aim to poker game and antes all he's got.
He played 'em tight and came out right, one thousand skins his pot!
Now feeling tall he bets it all, excitement fills the room;
When comes an eight to fill his straight, it spelled the others doom!

Now his command is fifty grand, the slot machine is loaded,
And with his luck - his fortune struck...the jack pot box exploded!
Twelve thousand bills in silver spills right out onto the floor,
With cup he scoops and then he scoots to roulette wheels for more!
His blood is hot he dares to spot his loot on blood red shade;
Around it swirls, the ball it twirls, 'til on the red it laid!
With one big grin and one more spin, it all went on the line,
And when it stops from table tops, comes five hundred thousand, nine!

While now in style and with his pile he wants just one more try;
To stake his stack and play black jack on hands an egg could fry.
With apparent gall he put it all on a hand with double split;
He rakes a lot, a $ million pot! when "Black Jack" comes a hit!
So he takes his load and hits the road, it's time to go back home;
But while enroute he met a tout, a pal he once had known.
Without hinder to the race track window, he bets the entire lot;
To himself he mused, "I just can't lose," as it goes on this long shot!

He dreamed of fame to win his aim; to have no more appall;
But his horse was passed which came in last, and this guy just lost it all!
But a lesson learned is a blessing earned in avoiding this kind of hit;
Is taking your bread while you're ahead and do a "lickety de split"
So at his house when asked by spouse, "How did you do my sweet?"
And from him follows, "I lost the two dollars, Is there anything here to eat?"

ONE LIFE TO LIVE

High levels of cholesterol for many of us are a very serious problem. I went on a diet program in 1985, immediately after heart surgery to combat my situation, although it wasn't diagnosed quite as serious as that, but of having smoked many years ago.

Through the next 10 years I practiced the usual "No cholesterol diets," no red meat, no eggs, no cheese, etc. until I had to have it lowered medically. My cholesterol had risen to an undesired level. The following short verse, "One Life To Live," is my way to poke a little fun at this really very serious situation.

ONE LIFE TO LIVE

One coffee for breakfast, one piece of toast, one water for vitamin pill;
everything else I love the most, experts have claimed will kill!
'Cause out of control is cholesterol, the clogging is doing me in.
They say this effect will take its toll unless I begin this trend:

No omelets with cheese, with bacon or ham, hominy and easy fried eggs.
No biscuits, no pork, no corn beef spam, oh, how my hunger begs!
No butter, no bagels or waffles real hot, or dunkin' a chocolate doughnut
in a coffee pot with cream a lot, or jam on a plate piled up.

But only one coffee, one toast and pill, is breakfast that I take in.
This is suppose to last me until-- I reach dinner, and then:
No mayonnaise, no crackers, no frenchy fries, no roast beef or any red meat;
no cookies or cakes or pizza pies, only one fish to eat.

No salt on the fish, no sweet'ning the tea, no desserts, no peanuts or beer.
"This hunger is taking its toll on me, and it's not cholesterol I fear!"
No sauces or spices for 'tators that's hot, just down 'em pure simple and plain.
"Will someone pass me the dish I got? Oh! I'll never go hungry again!"

But only one 'tator, boiled fish not fried, is all of the dinner I ate;
at supper time if I'm still alive I'll have this food on my plate:
One salad, one tea, which is sugar free, with two slices of whole wheat bread.
If I don't go down with a clogged artery, from starvation they'll find me dead!

❖❖❖❖❖

SILLY SENILITY

Well, it happened again today! As I visited the mall I thought I saw someone I knew, but I couldn't place his face. It seems to happen a lot these days. I hope it's not too serious a disease! I think they call it old age! However, I'm not going to worry about it. I'm doing what I suggest in my poem, "Silly Senility." I'm going to ask them who they are!

SILLY SENILITY

Memory has a funny way of fading to a blur,
many things remembered are not like they were.
I see a lot of faces from the past they will come,
without a name in mind to match with anyone!

Sometimes I watch my TV of some old movie show,
and often I see someone I know that I know,
but cannot seem to place them in that film made long ago.
Now it was only yesterday while passing time a way,
when I saw one in the mall whom I could not recall
as we walked along the hall.

I couldn't place his face when he went by me
in haste with nothing said at all!
And when I'm looking back to see
if he was looking back at me, I could see
him looking back at me to see
if I was looking back to see if he was looking back at me.

It was as I thought it was, I thought it so because:
He was thinking my same thought, and looking back, brought pause!
I suppose it was the case, he couldn't place my face,
so in our brain our memories strain;
maybe our paths will cross again,
and if they do I'll stop to greet, shake his hand when we meet,
ask his name and then I'll see just whose face is bugging me!

❖❖❖❖❖

SINCE WHEN

It's been some time since Ben has seen his twin named Ken.
They were the age of ten when they departed then.
The twins Mom, named Lynn, and Dad, whose name is Flynn,
Were separated when twins life would start to blend,

But, Ben went with Father Flynn, who used to bend rims
At Mercedes Benz-- but lost his job since then!
Mother Lynn took Ken, the other twin,
And moved around the bend next to Flynn's brother, Tim,

Who doesn't claim Flynn as kin, 'cause Flynn fills his glass to the brim
With favorite "Gilbys Gin", downs it with a winning grin,
And to Tim--This does offend! Mother Lynn spins a cotton gin,
While Ken, the twin, tends the bin.

They both are fond of neighbor Tim, or Uncle Tim to Ken,
Who lives next door to them. Ken and Ben now want to spend
More time with Lynn and Flynn, asking them to mend their trend
With message they now send.

It's been too long since Lynn and Flynn and brother Tim, their kin,
Gathered twins, Ben and Ken and all shared Love within.
Now Flynn and Lynn, divorced in sin and did not church attend,
Says chances slim but will amend their lives with hopes to blend.

I guess it's time to put an end to all this non-sense spin...
So let's get Lynn and Flynn, Ben and Ken to see them back again,
Then ask Tim to visit them without his usual whim-
And maybe then they'll all intend to make amends as friends,
Then strive to mend and all will win.
AMEN!! WHEW!

THE INMATE AND THE FLY

A man was sent to prison found guilty of a crime,
he stole what wasn't "His'en", for that he's doing time.
While there he comes defiant, so he's placed in solitaire,
where nothing was reliant brought anguish and despair.
He thought he may go crazy, or at worse, he could die;
when across his cell-so hazy, he saw a little fly.
With hands so soft and very quick, he caught that little fly;
to teach him how to do a trick as time goes passing by.
It was his aim to then preserve his mind and sanity,
to try and keep a steady nerve until they set him free.
Now thirteen years have gone on by with inmate in control;
and many tricks he taught the fly, one was to make him roll,
and also trained that fly to sing, lie down and play dead,
trained him how to dance and swing, and stand upon his head.
The inmate came to be real glad and proud of his long deed,
of this special fly he had, and too, from prison- freed!

The two became close bonded friends, this inmate and the fly,
and now they're free to make amends, they bade the prison bye.
But out of the iron clad prison gate they don't go very far;
because he stopped to celebrate at nearby drinking bar.
He entered with a glowing face and strolled up to the bar,
removed the fly from his suitcase to show his special "star".
Then at the bar he sounded with firm and eager call,
To the waiter who had rounded some glasses down the hall.
Said he: "Hey waiter! Come see our special act, you won't believe your eye!"
And the waiter came... with one quick smack, and Squashed that little Fly!!!
Now there's a moral to this story which happens all the time;
That man can reach his fondest glory creating something fine;
To gain success in life's hard strain, then see it quickly-down the drain!
And man is also like that fly, so small and innocent;
to accomplish deeds that odds defy...with results so quickly spent!!

❖❖❖❖❖

JO, JOE, BO, BOW AND ARROW

Now here is Bo and his girl Jo,
whom he loves so dear;
Now Jo calls Bo her lasting beau,
and Bo calls Jo his dear.

Now Bo asks Jo if she wished to go
to hunt with Bo for deer.
Bo asks Joe, who like Jo,
is Bo's best friend so dear.

So here goes Jo, Bo, and Joe
to hunt with bow for deer.
They all love the arrow and bow,
a sport they love so dear.

But Bo, like Jo, but unlike Joe,
managed to spot a deer,
Bo fired the arrow from his bow
and missed by ten feet clear!

Jo told Joe to keep down low
while she took her shot to go;
and while she missed the fleeing doe,
she shot her beau named Bo!

TO BEAR KNOT

It's not easy to teach a bear how to tie a knot!
Although your hands may be bare, the bear's paws are not.
Just bear in mind the bear's paws are full of furry hair;
This very reason is because he is a grizzly bear!

For him, the bear, to tie this knot is more than he can bear,
Because its fingers he has not, but claws to claw his lair.
Now here you have to bear some hope that the bear must bear in mind,
That to tie a knot with rope is not as good as twine.

To tie a knot is worse with string, besides string does not rhyme!
So, you must always bear in mind that your bare hands cannot
Tie knots with any fishing line of any simple knot.
And be aware that the bear cannot bear in mind,
That this is all you can bear with line of any kind.

So why bother any bear with tying knots at all?
The bear doesn't really care. And on you, all burdens fall!

❖❖❖❖❖

OLD TIMER

While I was strolling down the street one bright and sunny day,
skipping along with happy feet upon my merry way,
I came upon this gentleman rocking in his chair,
fanning with a make-shift fan to stir the humid air.

He looked to be 'bout ninety three with hair as white as snow,
and he cupped his eyes so he could see, and his skin was wrinkled so!
He cupped his ear so he could hear when I went up to speak,
and shook his hand when I got near, but how his grip was weak!

I shouted then, "How are you friend?" I wish you'd share with me,
the secret to the life you spend, and your longevity?"
In his feeble way he began to say: "This is how it is,
drink two six packs of beer each day along with six gin fizz!"

"Dance and dine with gals and wine, and gamble through the night,
and do not stop to whine or pine... keep going with all your might!"
Then I said to him: "That's some great trend, I think I'll try that too,
but do you mind my old dear friend, tell me how old are you?"
With an answer sly, and wishful eye, he said: "No I don't mind"
'cause today I'm celebrating my birthday, I'm Twenty-Nine!!"

❖❖❖❖❖

ALL ABOUT FISHING

Because of the nature of my work as a railroad brakeman, the opportunities were few to go fishing or play golf. However, upon my retirement I took up these two sports like wild fire in a wheat field. Although I came to do both very well, I certainly don't profess to be an authority on either. These following two poems only reflect my opinion, in a whimsical way, what I perceive them to be, and do not necessarily depict them as true.

"All About Fishing"
"All About Golf"

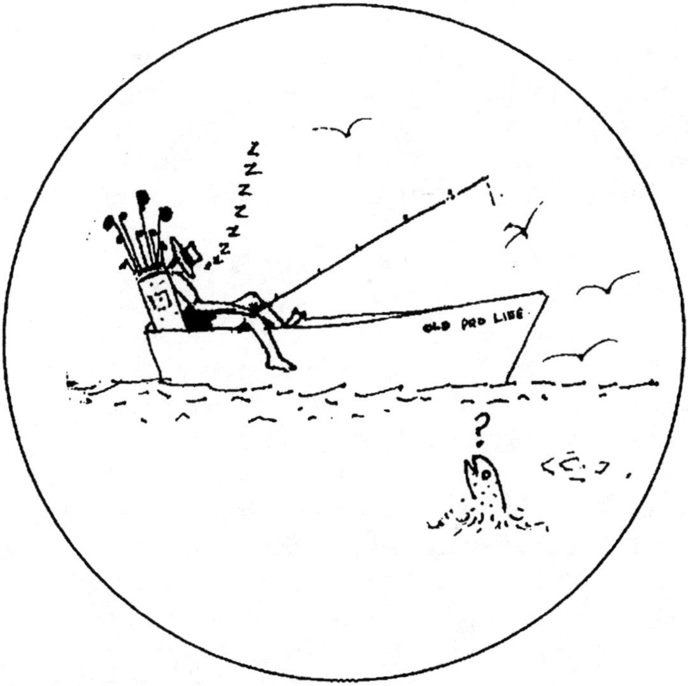

ALL ABOUT FISHING

Fishing is an exercise done for many years,
not for body building, but for strength between the ears!
And often times I wonder why all folks love to fish;
is there anything that's better, to fill another wish?

I'll put that question down to rest and not even try,
because I know there's nothing best--than a pan of fish to fry.
While many folks won't eat 'em, but love to reel 'em up-
well, they don't know what they're missing when it's time to fill their gut!

Fishing in a lake or stream is more than just plain luck--
--it's knowing where to take the boat without it getting stuck;
and one must know what bait to use, and that the fish are there,
or else he surely finds his cooler mighty bare!

We cast our lines out from the banks, or boat, or standing bridge...
we just can't get enough of this... until we fill the "fridge".
There are so many species of fish found everywhere;
and that's what makes the sport it is ... a challenging affair.

Now fishing is a science, and it's also just a game,
we can't decide on proper lures, 'cause none are made the same.
Now fishing is divided between one's luck and skill,
and if we practice both of these, there's sure to be a thrill;

but if you don't do either, you'll surely come to say:
"Just as I thought it would, the big one got away!"
A zeal to fish could do you in and mar your married life,
unless you take some time and spend it with your wife!

To fish is so relaxing with solitude to bear,
for when you're casting out your line---you cast away your fear.
Fishing isn't always kind, there's disappointments too;
'cause many hours go for naught while searching for a clue.

When you go out fishing, take the kids along;
for this will keep them off the street---just where
they don't belong!
It is a wise decision and the kids will get the "Bug"
and when they catch their fish...don't you forget to hug!

I really can't explain it all why people love it so;
fishing grips us to the bone with many tales to stow,
and can't begin to tell you folks of all the things I know,
for many fish have different names... too many waters flow;

but nothing can be better and nothing more sublime,
than something with a mighty tug 'a pulling on your line!
The mystery is so ecstatic- you wonder what you caught,
and this is what its all about... is what that moment brought.
I've said enough on fishing now, I'm heading for the links,
'cause golfing is my second love, to cure my ailing kinks!

❖❖❖❖❖

ALL ABOUT GOLF

This is a game played by the young and also by the old.
It doesn't matter if its hot, or even if its cold!
The game is just a honey, it humbles everyone.
It's played for skill, played for money, played for only fun.
But it's also played for exercise, at least some people say,
but when their "swing" is in demise, all hell has got to pay!
Winston Churchill had his say, I'll use his quote today:
"Golf is not effective way... propelling a little sphere;
uncontrollable all asway, to small holes that aren't near.
Instruments that we use are ill adapted too,
swinging them to just confuse, is not the thing to do!" (Unquote.)

Though what a way to spend a day, chasing a small white ball.
"Leave your woes at home" they say, "Play golf to answer call."
Then tee it up and take a stance and sight the long fairway,
wiggle and waggle with a dance... then miss it in a sway!
You teed it low 'cause wind was high, but then the wind died down...
your errant shot went all awry, to the woods and out of bound!
There comes a part of usual play, you'll find your ball in "rough";
"too many times" I must say: "can make this game play tough"
I found my ball in bunkered sand, I thought it reached the "green"...
I really do not understand, this game of golf is mean!

This game can also let you down or either lift you up,
but that depends on if you frown, or ball has holed the cup!
One more say about what's done, and that is: practice long,
and do it with an eye for fun and nothing will go wrong!
Now some people head out to the links for no particular reason...
they lost their love for bowling rinks...but now, its golfing season!!
They flock in numbers to the tee on every early morn,
some have tried to shun their fee, each day a cheaters born!
Some have shown no will for caring, they just get there in the way...
they only come for daily pairing to waste another day.
Some are ill and in dismay, and many are confused...
but they show-up anyway, good players feel abused!

I've seen 'em throw clubs all around and out into the water...
not even the ball they crowned... went out there any farther!
Once upon a short, first hole, a ball flew close to me.
Some guy had been so very bold to strike it from the tee.
Later, he said: "I'm in a fix and feeling blue, I'm told my wife is sick,
so can I play on through by you, so I can see her quick?"
Sometimes I think this game is grand, but you meet near every kind,
always watch it where you stand... especially from behind!
This is how it always is when e'er you play this game,
I would really be remiss if I didn't point some blame.
If we become too serious here, it ceases as a game
and results will bring much misery near... and that can be a shame!

The key is in our attitude, we strive to keep it good,
this will help us hit the ball with iron clubs or a wood.
And when we play as not a fool, we'll smack it very far,
and hit it straight when we stay cool and we will score at par.
I'd say more about this game that takes a lot of time--
but only few have reached a fame by playing golf sublime.
Golf is fun, but irritating if it gets the best of you,
so play the game without deflating and you'll love it through and
through.
I'll just close this prose by stating: "Golf was surely good for me,
while I had no special rating---I was in good company!"

That's golf folks!

❖❖❖❖❖

WHAT'S IN A NAME

Now everybody all have names, everything else does too,
so everyone should take the pains to find out which is who!
It never fails I must confess that when I'm waved upon;
it's always "Hey" on their address, or "Hi there" on the phone.

For many years I wondered why the folks just wouldn't say
my real true name which I rely instead, they called me "Hey!"
Even now, when I hear "Hi there!" I think they're calling me,
but then I guess it's better fare, than the name of "Do Hick-He."
There's "Thing-a-ma-jig" or "Whas-his-name"
along with "Thing-a-ma-bob," it's not intended to defame,
but an ego it will rob. There's "Ding-a-ling," " Do-lolly-pop,"
"Whacha-ma-callit," and "Do Dad,"
"Rink-a-dink," and "Boppety bop"
are some of the names we've had.

But I have to say there is a trend that people seem to show;
that even to some close by friend, my name, they still don't know.
Most precious thing we have on earth for with us mortals stay;
is our very name we got at birth, for everyone to say!
So if it's asking not too much, be a little more direct,
and use not labels or the such, but our true names we respect!

❖❖❖❖❖

ALL FOR THE THOUGHT

Strange things happen when you live way out and apart from the rest of the world.
Your heart wears out from a yearning bout when your thoughts get stuck on a girl!
He's a lonely guy who's lost away, and pines for a woman's care.
He spends some time every single day thinking of a maiden fair.

And he plans this day to go and look at the next small town away;
he needs a wife who can sew and cook, and help bail up the hay.
And his very first stop is a far away nook, ten miles to that farm house.
Once he's there he'll start to look for girl to be his spouse.

Now he leaves on foot 'cause there is no road; just nothing but woods around;
with a small canteen in a back pack load, he heads to the first small town.
He's only in the woods about a half a day before he comes to know;
that some where along the thick pathway, he forgot which way to go!

So he goes in circles for fifteen days, and all his supplies run out;
all he can do is hope and pray, that he'll find the proper route.
But in his plight he trudges on through every other nook and cove;
he's willed determined to overcome, for the sake of a woman's love.

After several more days, he's about wore out, no food, nor water for rinse,
but his eyes catch sight of an old milk cow there scratching on a barb wire fence!
He knew he'd found the first small town as he peered through his blood shot eyes,
at that first little shack that he has found, that sits there atop the rise.

With his legs now sprawled, he commences to crawl like a snake that's after a mouse.
With a parched out throat he attempts to call to that little old shanty house,
but his voice is low, 'cause his throat hurt so, and no one heard his cry,
but he set his sight on where to go, to the door steps that were nigh.

Well, he crawls to the porch, his throat is hoarse, lying prone, just a total wreck!
With very little strength, but just enough force to rap there upon the deck.
And a man inside, hurries outside to give this man a hand,
and he says with pride, "If you'll confide, I'll help you all I can."

And the wretched man could hardly speak, but he managed: "Do you have a daughter?"
and the farmer, with a voice less weak, said: "No, but I have food and water!"
And with that answer the poor man said: "My flame you cannot douse,
but my dear friend I'll ask instead, how far is the next farm house?"

Strange things happen when you live way out, and apart from the rest of the world.
Your heart wears out from a yearning bout when your thoughts get stuck on a girl!

❖❖❖❖❖

THE BALLAD OF STATUS QUO

"I had a hectic time last night," I told my wife close by.
"What on earth is ailing you?" She asked me to say why.
She wished to know about my woe, and this was my reply:
"I'll tell you dear what are the facts: my body's racked with pain,
My arm to thumb is deadly numb 'cause on them I have lain,
And cannot seem to find them now, ten minutes here in vain.
My foot is sorely aching from stumping toes last night-
On chair legs in the darkness that was hidden out of sight,
And the rest of night was restless from pain I had to fight!
Then, when upon that happening I woke you up my spouse,
With my sudden screams of shouting that filled the entire house,
A pain so powerful burning... a flame I could not douse.

My old stiff neck still hurts "cause of pillows stacked too high,
Like an old familiar feeling when I wore a suit and tie,
And these crinks which don't leave easy, leads a grown up man to cry!
And watching midnight movies made my eyes so sore and red...
Added sorrow to my torment and also aching head...,
And the morning looks no brighter as I dread it here in bed...
And my knees are swollen knobby like those on oak or pine--
Brought on by arthritis and tolled by length of time--
And all their use is adding to the ailments that I find.
My legs are also scrawny just like an old oak tree,
Crooked and bowed and pigeon toed, like any old legs can be,
But I will cope in entire hope with all my misery.

Now my back is bent with aging with years of taking toll,
And I dare not do no lifting, not even my fishing pole...
And up and down most of the night, I think I've caught a cold!
And all the pills and capsules I take for everything,
Should keep my body going with much relief from sting,
But I suspect as often... no hope they'll ever bring,
But you ask what's wrong with me my dear, so this I now relate;
All the things I've told to you are just some facts of fate;
But outside all I've spoken here, I Feel Absolutely Great!!!

❖❖❖❖❖

Our home is located next to an elementary school and it occurred to me recently just how happy most everyone seemed to be as I viewed them approaching the school. Of course there were many of the small ones showing some discontent, but my very short poem, "Back To School", reveals the true recipients of happiness.

BACK TO SCHOOL

Today's the day the kids return,
To some, the hour of gloom,
But others show a happy yearn
To fill their new class room.

But the happiest ones, I suspect,
Are their parents who are glad!
For summer long, the pool and deck
Have worn out Mom and Dad!

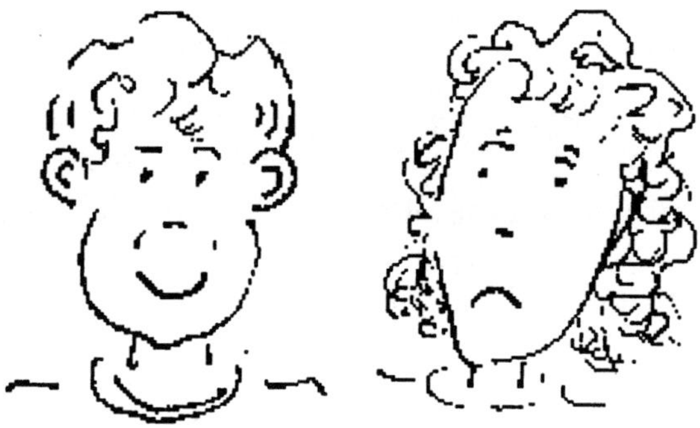

"THE DOVE"

In our lives at some point we'll see in our midst someone who "puts on heirs of being above it all", so to speak. These individuals seem to portray themselves as somewhat better than their peers.

These persons are generally the ones who only show at certain occasions, such as church on Easter, or perhaps some social function where they may want to further their cause.

These certain people should really have an opportunity to see themselves as others see them. So in my following poem, "The Dove", is my effort to do that.

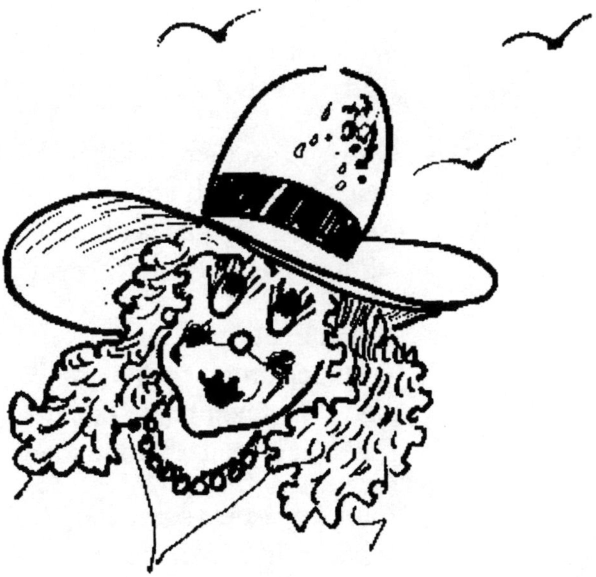

THE DOVE

It was on an Easter Sunday
In a busy city church,
Where some folks came to worship
In an effort there to search,

But in this congregation
Were some "high falootin" ones
Who came to show their garments
When ever Easter comes.

Now in the eyes of others
You don't know how you look
Until some realization shows
"You got your picture took"!

For sitting in that mass
Was a lady all agleam
With her bluish, blackish, lashes,
And her rosy facial cream.

Now she sat there "high and mighty"
Just a'peering all around,
As if the Lord had sent her
With her frilly bonnet crown

To captivate an audience
With performance Ala grand,
And send them home believing
She's the queen of wonderland.

But here there's something lacking
When you take the time to stop
To see upon her bonnet
A blackish, whitish spot!

Now it seems the only answer
Comes from heaven up above,
Where a sign of revelation came,
By droppings from a dove!!

❖❖❖❖❖❖❖❖

"IS IT TERMINAL?"

There is I believe a dreadful disease that's sweeping the earth and really can be devastating. I never had it but I might have thought a few times in my life that I had a symptom or two, but I fought it off until I could get back on the right track.

It's not really clear by the experts if it's contagious or inherited, but I tend to think it's a great deal of both. In my poem, "Is It Terminal?", clears up the facts about this disease.

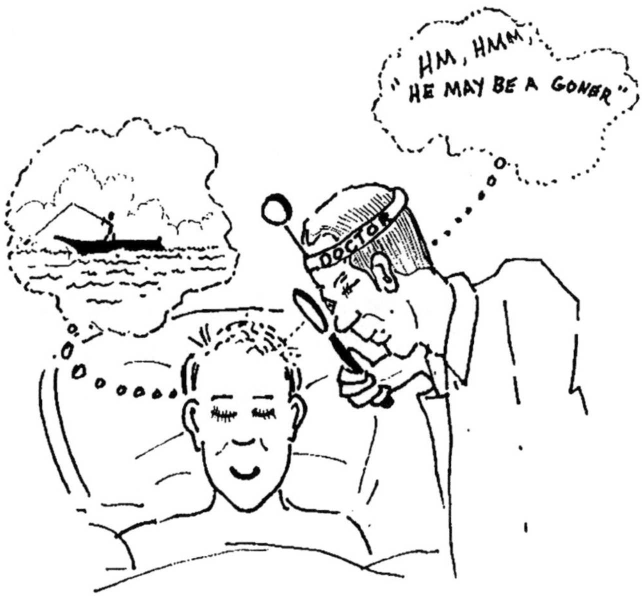

IS IT TERMINAL?

The worst disease that's known to man
Which experts came to know,
Is it grips a body like no ill can,
And makes a person slow.

With gender all it knows no bound,
It rots away their soul.
It shys away their peers around
As this illness takes its toll.

It affects all people on the earth,
It bleeds away their pride.
It robs away their inner mirth,
Its symptoms cannot hide.

The cure outlook for this disease
Remains a little hazy,
But ease is best when patients sees;
Their problem is they're LAZY!!.

❖❖❖❖❖❖❖❖

"THE RIGHT TEMPERATURE"

After review you may see a great deal of truth in my remedy for a long and lasting marriage. First, I must tell you that my wife Bobbie, and I have been married for 42 years and for a large portion of that time we both worked, usually at different times, so as the old saying goes, "absence makes the heart grow fonder" was in a large sense true in our case.

Secondly, we practiced the things described in my next verse, "The Right Temperature." So as not to give away too many secrets at once, I'll allow the following poem to do that.

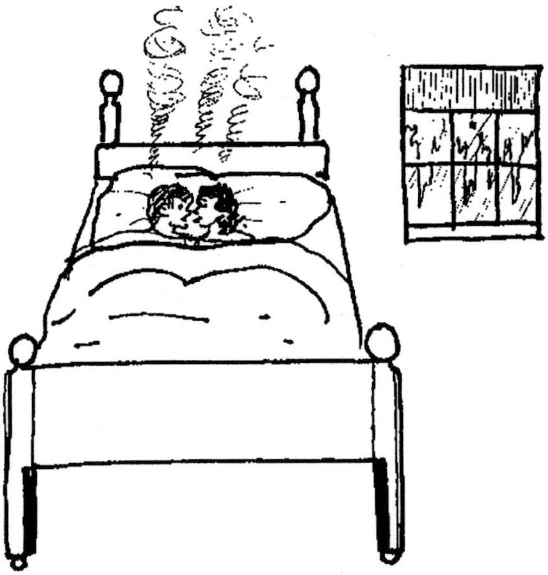

THE RIGHT TEMPERATURE

Now, I've been thinking
And I know it's true,
And it's how to manage
Your marriage through.

There's one thing certain
And two things sure,
You have to stay close
To work this cure:

First, you agree not to disagree,
Then look to see what the other one sees,
Then decree that you both agree,
Then live each day with this appease.

That's number one,
But I've only begun,
The next solution
Is the hardest one.

You have to listen,
It's your mind one seeks,
And don't plan your comments
While the other one speaks!

Hear what is said
Then give your reply,
And then you'll see
Things eye to eye.

Now last, not least,
And the best of all
Is turn down the thermostat
That's on your wall.

You turn it down
When you go to bed,
And it saves your light bill
That you dread,

But it does something else
You need to know.
It guarantees a closeness
For you in stow!

For if outside
It's cold as ice
And you both are cuddled up
Really nice,

This builds up a bond
When you two clasp,
And this will surely
Make your marriage last!

❖❖❖❖❖❖❖❖

"ALWAYS CHANGE"

Due to our life styles in a capitalistic world our daily endeavor is handling money in one form or another. Although I realize it will never happen, I would seriously be a strong supporter of eliminating the penny from our currency system.

Now if you stop to think about it, the penny doesn't really do anything constructive, but on the other hand, it creates a lot of inconvenience and loss of time, both for the public and the treasury department.

In the following verse, "Always Change", I describe my version of the situation and what I hope would correct it.

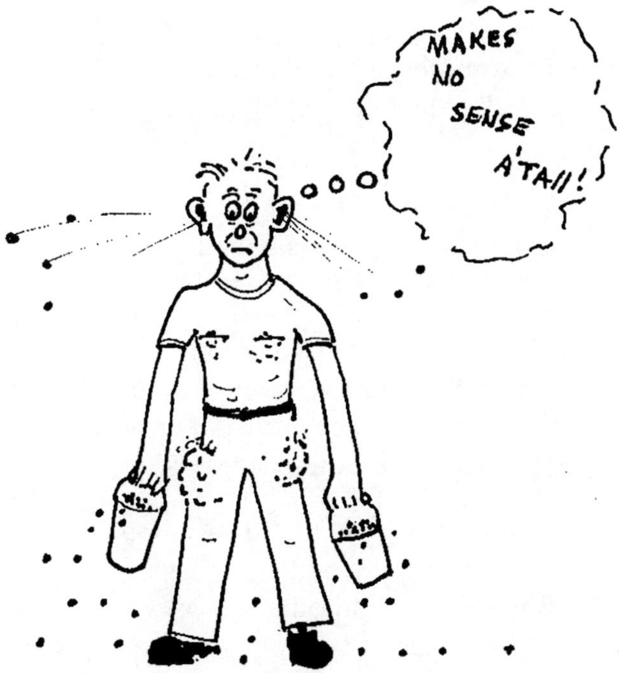

ALWAYS "CHANGE"

It is a trend I hope will end,
The one that deals with "change",
The jingling kind that builds with time,
But still no value claims.

This special change that "feds" could make
Is do away with pennies,
"For everybody's gracious sake
The pennies must diminish!"

If all the pennies that they mint
Were melted all away,
It would do away with trouble spent
And headaches and dismay.

'Cause pennies often load us down,
Our pockets always fill,
They're everywhere they can be found,
For all around they spill!

And when you go to shop around
You'll see upon the signs,
A very clever price is bound
Which always ends in nines!

Form zero-nine to ninety-nine
This item cost is plain,
That what it means is what it deems,
That pennies is your change!

So now they go in overflow
In every cup and jar,
Within a vase, in some suitcase
Or floor board of your car!

In pocket book, the dining nook,
The sofa and your chair,
In all ash trays, in window bays,
And on the way upstairs.

On table tops, in many spots
These pennies all are spied,
They'll ever stay in all our way--
Until this trend has died!

It would be nice, it would suffice
To round it to one dollar--
'Twould be no "change" to tax our brains,
And be the trend to follow.

❖❖❖❖❖❖❖❖

"NEED OF REPAIR"
"MECHANIC IN THE SKY"

The following verse, "In Need of Repair", reminds us of how important it is for us to get our belongings inspected or parts repaired as we travel on this road of life.

These inspections and repairs should be done often so as not to run into some real serious problems down the road. The next verse, "Mechanic In The Sky", merely indicates the best place to go for these repairs and inspections.

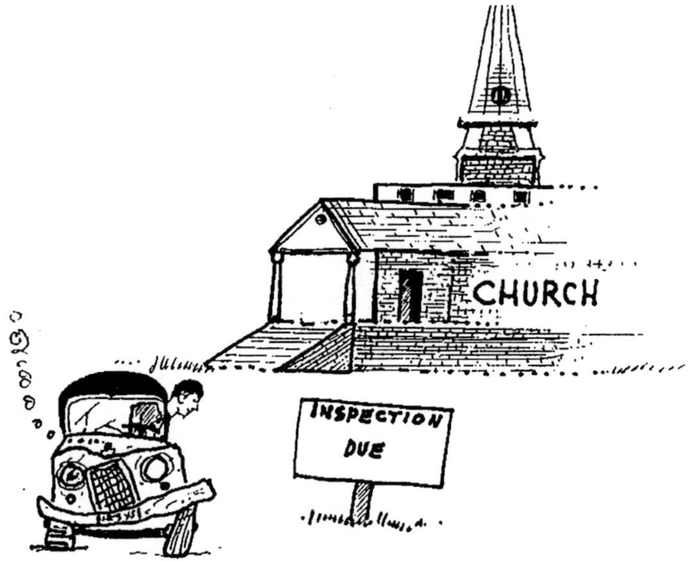

IN NEED OF REPAIR

I'm stranded by the lone roadside,
My motor just conked out.
My route has been a rocky ride
Of many miles about.

I've been driven, pushed, and tampered with,
And left out in the cold.
I've given all that I can give,
My parts are getting old!

I need a new replacement valve,
My fuel is all burnt out.
The trouble that I am facing now
Is leaving me in doubt.

My battery needs recharging and
Its strength is mighty weak.
It's given all that I demand,
It's reached the final peak!

If I could get another coil,
More sparkling would revolve,
And there would be less tedious toil,
And problems would resolve.

A brand new starter would begin
To start my life anew;
And bring my strength to go again
With freshness I once knew.

It's all these parts I need thus far,
The reason is you see;
They're not really for my car,
These repairs are all for me!

❖❖❖❖❖❖❖❖

MASTER MECHANIC IN THE SKY

Our bodies, like cars or old guitars,
All three need a check some time,
But it takes someone to make it all run
By tuning our life real fine!

But we should inspect the ones that check,
To see that we don't get rooked;
So we pick the best to complete this test
And not the one who's crooked.

So if your motor whines and your cam shaft binds,
Then you need a check throughout;
For a fuel that soiled to a tank that boiled,
To find what it's all about!

Now don't show your face down at Satan's place,
'Cause he did your work before;
For he's the crook, from your life who took
The strength from your motor's core.

And he's the one who allowed it to run,
Causing the over heat;
And he burned your wires with his careless fires,
Which he tangled up in a heap!

So upon this time find an ace who's fine,
Who works with his morals high.
A mechanic fair with a sound repair,
Who will make your energy spry.

I've heard of one, one of the best, bar none!
And He works from His shop on high.
So if you got any amp that needs revamp,
Look for Him in the sky!

❖❖❖❖❖❖❖❖❖

"SHAD ANYONE?"

Seafood is a delicious dish, and one of the most popular game fish is called "shad." It is also one of the tastiest that can be caught, but shad also has a reputation for being the "boniest" of them all.

Now there are several ways in which to prepare this wonderful fish to obtain the best flavor possible, and in my verse "Shad, Anyone?" depicts the method many people have described as being one of the best ways.

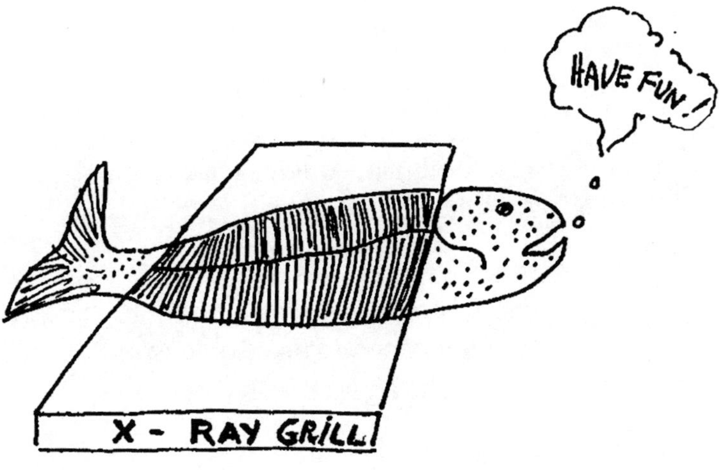

SHAD, ANYONE?

A gamely fish within the sea,
Its name is called a "shad";
No better catch will ever be
With all the fun you had!

There's always been a lot of say
On how to cook this fish.
A boney "shad" you can't fillet
With all his bones like this!

To take this fish upon a dish
And in the oven bake;
Would be against your very wish
For eight hours it would take.

To fry him in a frying pan
Would be too awful quick;
The food just wouldn't taste as good,
And there's still the bones to pick!

It is the mood with this seafood
Oh how to best prepare.
It's understood to take some wood
And make a plank with care---

---The "shad" you fix with spicy mix,
And on this plank attach,
Place on a grill, below you fill
With wood and strike a match---,

Then roast the "shad" until its cured
With ample time to cook;
With best results to be assured
You give it one more look---,

---Then with the plank where this fish lies
You swing a mighty crank,
And hurl that "shad" far to the skies---,
---Then eat the spicy plank!!

"THE SPECKS"

Many of us already wear glasses for vision problems, so to you who are in this situation may be reminded of all these small pestering things that occur from time to time, but I can't imagine anyone else having the complexity with them as I do. Maybe I've never really gotten used to them!

To other folks, this following verse titled "Specks" may be in some ways an alert on what to expect. In any event, my sympathy, my hope, my regards, my sorrow, goes out to all who have to rely on them. But in the "Specks" I'm poking a little fun at it.

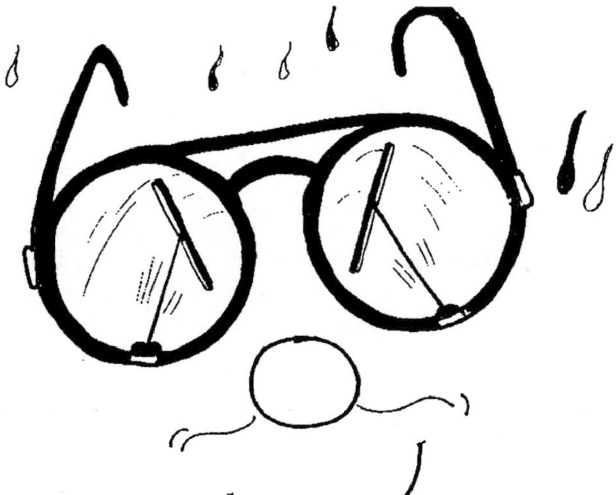

THE SPECKS

For those of you who aren't there yet
You're in for much surprise,
For as you age you'll need to get
Some glasses for your eyes.

For 10 years now I've had my pair
And they are one big pain,
Not in my eyes,...but you know where!
I'll try here to explain:

These "peepers", when I have them on
Will fog or steam right up,
Especially when I'm here at home
And drinking from a cup,

Or going out into the rains,
Or working up a sweat.
Moisture brings the biggest pains
That I've encountered yet!

And still there's other problems here
Like when they're in their case,
Because they're always lost somewhere,
Just where, I cannot place.

Or when I bend to tie my shoes
They always quickly fall
Upon the floor to get abused,
The glass, the frame and all.

And there were times I oft' forgot
And left them in the car,
To look for days around the lot
Just wondering where they are.

But after all they're what I need,
I'll try hard not to pout,
'Cause with these "specks," I have to read,
"Which someday you'll find out!"

"GIZMO"

Of course we're all aware of the population explosion, the tremendous surge of traffic upon our roads and highways, and the increase of these traffic lights that control our intersections. Now, I can't speak for others, but it certainly seems to me that I'm just catching too many lights that turn red, and they appear to start this change with the caution yellow flashing on just about the time I reach the 50 yard mark, which of course guarantees that I sit for that red light through its entirety.

Now this strange phenomenon began years ago and is still in progress today, in fact, it appears to worsen as does the traffic. I'm convinced that something must be causing it, so with all seriousness aside I explain in the following verse, "Gizmo", as to what I think it is.

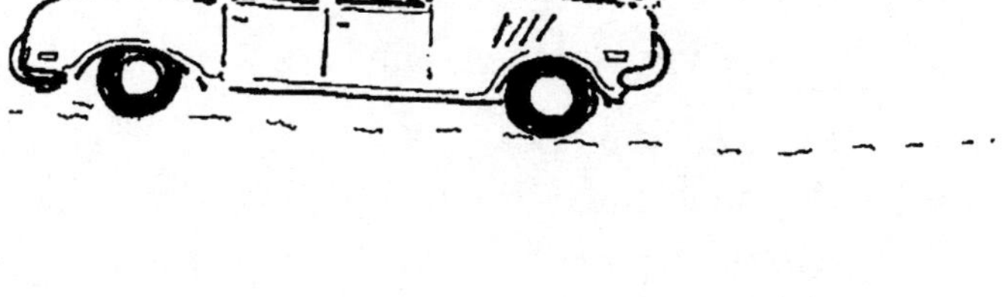

GIZMO

There is a little "gizmo" thing,
I think, on my car hood,
I guess a tool
Invisible.
It's not one understood!

I've often tried to locate it
But much to no avail,
Yet there it sights
The traffic lights,
It's never known to fail.

For while I drive in traffic's flow
In days, or 'lone at nights,
It always seems
To change the beams
As I approach those lights.

The strangest thing is what it brings,
It always turns 'em red,
And I've never seen
It turn 'em green,
It's always red instead!

So in my woe I watch the glow
Of every "red" in town,
But on I'll drive
And I will strive
To keep my temper sound.

Tho' see him not
He's in a spot,
In case there is a wreck,
This thing "gizmo"
Is first to go---
---And break his little neck.!

❖❖❖❖❖❖❖❖❖

The following two verses, "A Case of Mistaken Identity" and "Prophecy?", are nonsensical pieces designed only to bring a smile.

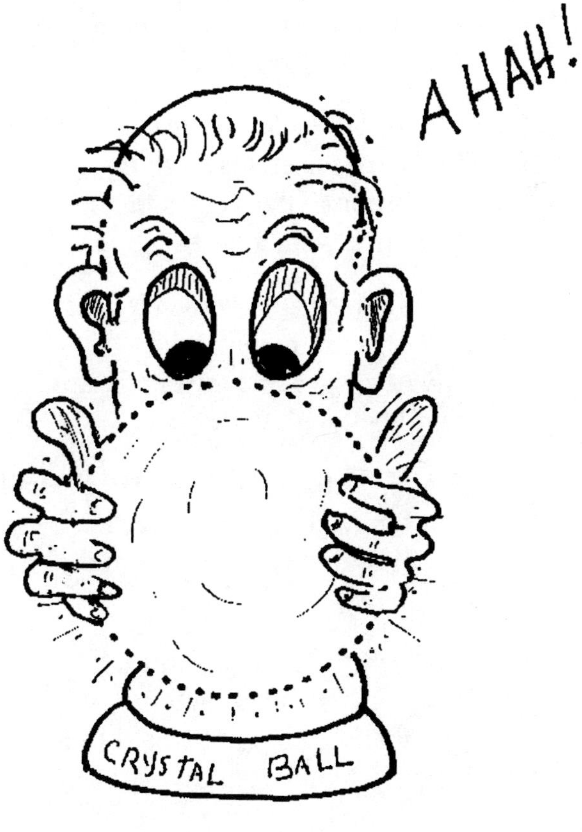

A CASE OF MISTAKEN IDENTITY

We play a team that's mighty mean,
This football power house.
They swamp their foe with all they know,
Each man's a lousy louse.

We despise these guys and I surmise
We'll tangle when we meet.
We'll find a way to make them pay
And trounce them in defeat.

So comes the day for our big fray,
But here's the strangest thing,
The uniforms that they had on,
Like ours, were gold and green.

Now in this game with colors same
It's hard to tell who's who;
And here we came to fill our aim,
It will be tough to do.

Now the referees' call to kick the ball
And I'm ready to make the catch;
It comes to me and I'm off in flee
In this ferocious match!

I have the ball and down I fall
With tacklers piled on top,
And I'm in a kink but what I think
Is a very tempting plot,

For there beneath that ton of heap,
Like twins our colors blend,
And in my face I cannot place
Just whose is this rear end!

Below this mix I sight some sticks,
I think I'll poke his butt!
I'll teach this swine to be more kind,
I'm going to be more tough.

So without ado I shoved it through
And drove the splinter home;
There was a cry that rang on high,
That reached to kingdom come.

And now out there most everywhere,
Men's hearts are stout and glad;
But mine is wane from all the pain,
It was my behind I stabbed!!

❖❖❖❖❖❖❖❖

PROPHECY ?

I'm a pessimist? Is that what people
say?
Well, I am so surprised!
I didn't know they felt that way.
I thought I prophesied!

Although I am to some extent,
'Cause good thoughts mix with bad,
But either way a high percent
Of accuracy I've had.

I've learned to see the little things
That give results away,
Maybe my experience brings
Some truth in what I say.

It's just a trend that I got in
When I became retired.
It is a blend that comes within
Of thoughts that are required.

What I do, in my mind, review,
Realize some past event.
If results come through, this is my clue,
And it will be my hint.

If I get this feeling I once knew
Of a "picture that I paint".
And if it looks too good for true,
Then true it usually aint!!

Here's a sample I'll explain;
I once played games of ball,
And in a game where good luck came,
Appears when I recall.

This thought will click, and I'll predict,
Based on outcome of that game.
If I contradict the team I pick,
Results will be the same.

Now I advise to all the wise
Don't try my method here,
'Cause I surmise that you realize,
That none of this is clear!

❖❖❖❖❖❖❖❖

"OUT OF CONTROL"

Due to modern technology, todays television sets all have those small hand controls that changes the sound, channels, etc, and I wonder if anyone else has the same problem I do in keeping up with the thing. In the following verse, "Out of Control" accurately depicts my experience with it.

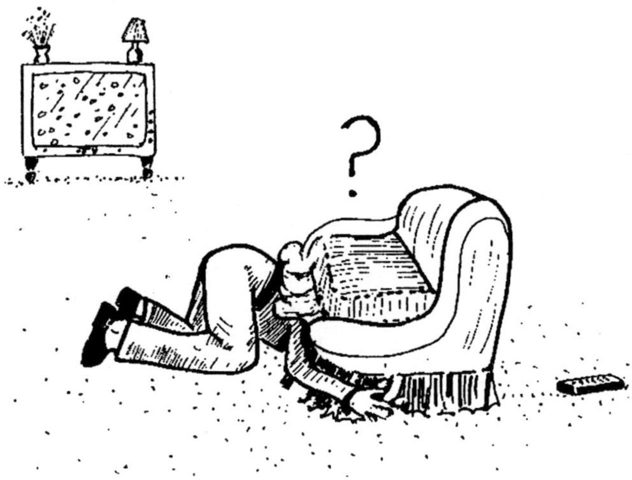

OUT OF CONTROL

I have a little hand control
That goes to my TV,
And somewhere in this world
I know it surely has to be,

For every time I put it down
It seems to disappear,
And though I know it isn't so,
It flees right in thin air!

I know it has no legs to walk,
Nor eyes to see to hide,
But every time I lay it down
Right there beside my side,

It finds a way to steal away
Before my very eyes,
And I look around, it can't be found,
All logic it defies.

I've even tried to tie a string
Around my neck to hold
This testy, small evasive thing
So it can be controlled!

But often then for reasons thin
It seems to get away,
And why it's so I just don't know,
And this goes on each day!

But it's been found in many spots,
I'll only name a few:
My recliner pouch, beneath the couch,
Under its pillows too.

On the floor, behind the door,
And under grandfather's clock,
In our bookcase, down in a vase,
And in a kitchen crock.

Down in the seat or in the pleat
Of my reclining chair.
The mantle top, the floor, a cot,
And sofa's lower flair.

The TV top, the fridge a lot,
(This one, often found!)
And I need that thing for me
To bring some sanity to the sound
(And to the sight as well!).

❖❖❖❖❖❖❖❖

"ONE DRINK TOO MANY"

The following verse "One Drink Too Many", is what I imagine one might say should he have one too many. It also may be a good reminder what not to do on many occasions such as birthday or New Year's Parties.

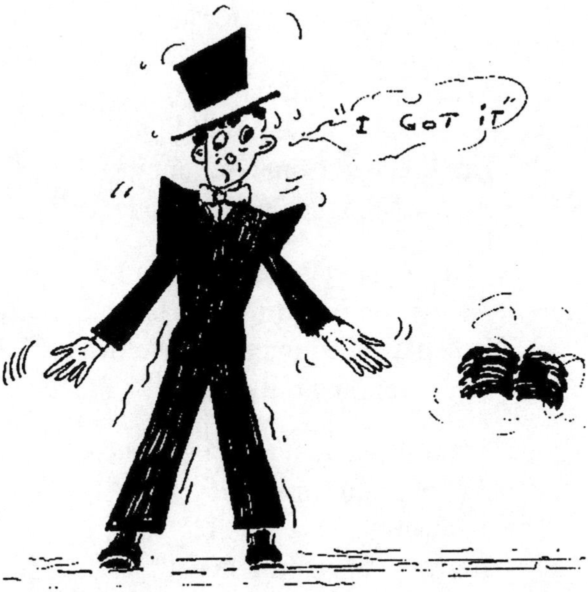

ONE DRINK TOO MANY

I'm dining out for breakfast
In a foreign, local bar,
When policemen stop to tell me
Just who it is I are!

It seems a strange thing happened
In the busy street last night
Where a hair piece went a flappin'
As it blew around in flight.

The policemen want to find out
Everything I sight,
So they can trace the where 'bout
Of a toupee that took flight.

I remember well what happened,
Although my memory's blurred,
But I'll keep from overlapping
As I tell them what occurred:

"The night was dark and shiny
As the sun was dimming bright;
When a naked man with clothes on
Came running out of sight!"

"And when he ran by near me
About 2 blocks aways;
The wind that wasn't blowing,
Blew off his bald toupee!"

"And when I helped to fetch it,
It stopped which I flew past,
And a bare-head man with hat on
Walked running for it fast!"

"When the wind stopped really blowin'
And the toupee had deceased,
A bare-foot boy with shoes on
Stood sitting on this piece."

"Now the bare-foot boy with shoes on
Just would not give it back--
To the naked man with clothes on
Who was trying to retract."

"Now I can say without a word,
I've lied the honest truth,
This folly really is absurd--
I'll stake my last VERMOUTH!!"

DIET MY WAY

So, you want to do a diet
And you don't know how to start?
Well, here's my way to try it
And I hope you will take part.
First, on every morn
When you open up your eyes,
You look upon your mirror form
The minute that you rise.

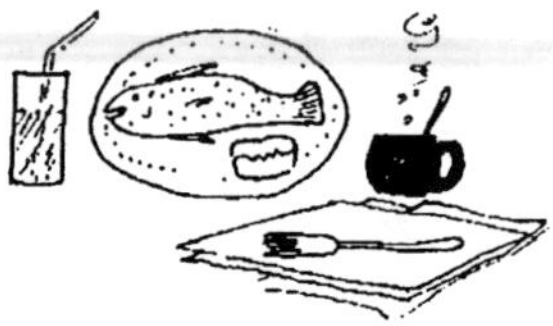

Now gaze upon your body
And evaluate your size,
If the sight reveals you're shoddy
Or in some great demise,
Then instead of morning toddy,
Do a daily exercise!

And do these calisthenics friend
With outlook that is wise,
You do them in your house but spend
Some time beneath the skies.
Where you do a lot of walking here
Each day with longer strides.
If the action is your highest gear,
You will lose it in the thighs!

But now please take another look,
I think you will surmise,
That your habits in the dining nook
Will come as no surprise.

For you need to cut your eating down
In order to survive,
And that means smaller portions found
In all your food supplies.

So breakfast now will find you
Perhaps with wishful sighs,
Because the morning meal that's few,
Is a portion that decries
Of one small bowl of bran buds
That hardly satisfies;
But you need these fiber grubs
So your system will revise.

So now it's time for dinner
Where you have the largest eyes,
But fish there is a winner
But it often brings out "whys".

But you have to stay in training
And do what you despise,
So you eat all your fish, retaining
The secret to down size.

Now supper is the time that brings
The best and greatest prize,
A great big bowl of salad greens
Where all the nutrients lies.

They eliminate the lows you frown,
And bring about the highs.
By now you are reducing down,
And saying last good-byes
To all the weight that you were bound
On all you gals and guys!

❖❖❖❖❖❖❖❖

There came a time in my life when I honestly tried to take stock of my life and get on some track that would take me in a different direction. I do pray and believe that I should try to live as close to the Golden Rule as I can. The following poems are my prayers.

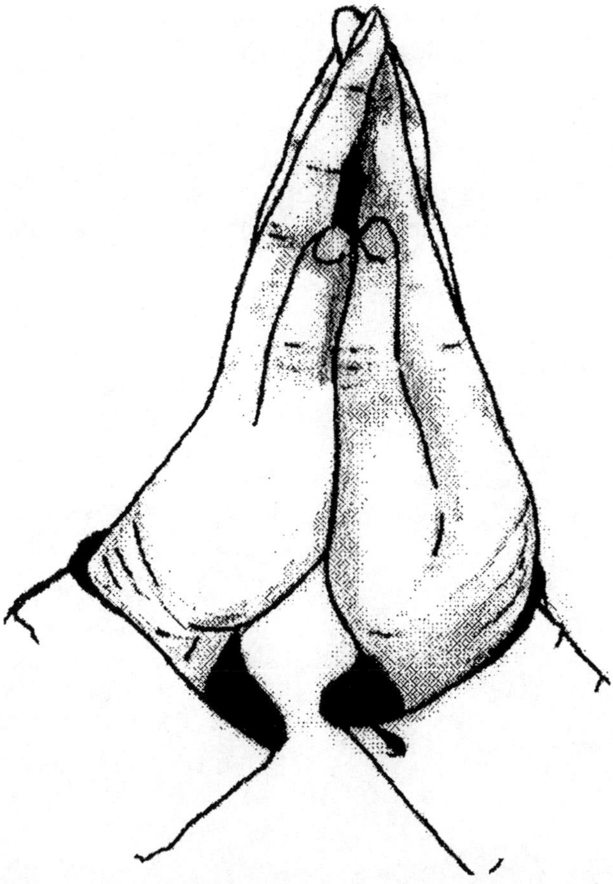

I'LL FOLLOW THIS RIVER

I'll follow this beautiful river,
A spirit within me glows;
With heart and mind I hope to find
The blessings God bestows.

I'll follow this beautiful river,
I'll follow these waters free,
And on the way I'll shout and pray
"I'm on to glory be!"

I'll follow this beautiful river,
Upon its tide I go;
To journeys end where waits my friend,
'Tis Jesus Christ I know.

I'll follow this beautiful river
With hope that lingers on,
He's there for me to set me free
And lead me to my home.

❖❖❖❖❖

BEST FRIEND

No vast fortune have I made,
Nor any claim to fame;
No honor, parade, or serenade
Or credit to my name.

Just a simple passer-by
That walks amongst the throng.
No special friends do I rely
Of those I pass along.

Just a face among the crowd
Of many wandering sheep.
With those I hope to be endowed
By God, His love I keep.

I may not walk with mortal friend,
But not alone I go,
No other voice do I depend
Save one I only know!

'Tis Jesus, by me walking
Along with every step.
'Tis Jesus, my friend we're talking ,
'Tis He that I accept!

❖❖❖❖❖

MY PRAYER

Lord, come lift me up and bring me
strength to face all problems here;
for peace of mind, with joy sublime,
erases all my fear.

You are my Savior, my reformer
and redeemer too;
so with your ever lasting love,
my life will start anew!

Dear Lord I pray, to thee I say:
I'm humble as can be;
come be my guiding light today
and live your life in me.

You are my faith, my hope and peace,
my life and true salvation.
Your very presence in my heart
instills a firm foundation.

So now dear Lord I give my thanks
for everything I own,
and everything you've done for me
and family, save none.

And now dear Lord I beg of You
to hear my words today,
for what I ask is in Your name,
in Jesus Christ I pray!

Amen.

THE MASTER'S VOICE

'Tis morning, I wake with solemn care from sleep with much dismay,
For I dreamed about a boat somewhere out on a water way.
It all was stark and all was dark as black as ace of spades,
No sight or light, not one small spark, just silence and the waves.
I squirmed and groped in some small boat I paddle with my might.
My clinging hope to stay afloat, and keep the craft upright.
I had a thought that as I fought, the waves around me tossed--
That I was on the open sea where I was surely lost!
About, abound, where darkness found a frightful stillness there;
'Twas so profound, no sight or sound while struggling in despair!
So for my life I shook in strife while coping woeful bind,
'Cause there was I in dreadful lie,...I dreamed I'm deaf and blind!
'Twas one nightmare too hard to bear, the scene that frightened so...
In striving there in desperate fear in search of where to go,
But I began to wonder then if this was just a sign,
Of how good life has really been--and how it's been so kind.
While suffering on that stormy sea in fright and fight out there,
A sweet soft voice astounded me and suddenly I could hear!
Those words, they came so very low and yet, they sounded clear:
"Be not in dismay or woe, there's nothing here to fear.
My will and love I now bestow, and with you I am near."
That lit the night with cast of light, my heart began to soar,
For God, His might, brought forth my sight and faith forevermore!
The ocean's crown then settled down with calm that crept the sea,
And when I cast my eyes around, a shore was plain to see,
For on my right, appeared a site to which I set to oar;
For now I see with precious sight a brilliant golden shore.
I lost all pain when once again His voice came very strong;
"You'll make it to that promised land where nothing will be wrong."
'Twas just a dream while there asleep, but know it was God's voice,
To bring me to him closer keep and in my soul rejoice!
And now the wake-up time is here I've opened up my eyes,
To me believing things are clear of facts I now realize,
That there are folks in their sad world born deaf and cannot see;
But the master speaks to them, behold! Just as he did to me.
But their ordeal is very real, mine, was only dreaming,
Never the less God does instill in all, a special meaning!

❖❖❖❖❖

FORGIVING

Dear God above, with all Your love
You gave Your son to me;
a friend in deed, my soul in need,
He died to set me free.

Christ braved the cross and took the loss
To save us all from sins,
We must believe as we conceive
His love that never ends.

With special goals to save our souls;
Great wonders to perceive!
So let us all be more like Him
And give what we receive.

Amen.

❖❖❖❖❖

LIFE'S WEARY HIGHWAY

Over this rocky road we tread, down the trails of life we trod--
through the pitfalls that we dread, searching for our God.
Beyond the mountains and the sea, a rainbow to the sky,
a heavenly path to glory-be; a place where angles fly...

Where, in that land, a peaceful place, we all meet in tomorrow;
so follow that rainbow with all your pace to freedom from all
sorrow.
If we show dear God our trust and pray with our true love,
He is always here to guide us - through that pathway up above.

❖❖❖❖❖

THANKSGIVING

I thank You Lord for all the days that I have seen on earth.
I thank You now for all the ways You show Your mighty worth.
I thank You too for all my strength which surely came from You,
And thanks again for this big lift, the power that sees me through.
I give my thanks for when I see I've been the lucky one;
While in this life where best is free, and God's own will is done!
I thank you Lord for being here in many times of strife.
You brushed away the ills and fear that came upon my life.

I thank You now for all the time when I was filled with glee.
The tolling of the bells that chime, meant your life had entered me.
I thank You for another cause, you wash away my sin;
It's done by Your abiding laws and love that has no end!
I thank you now for all my kids and also my dear wife.
I've been up and down the skids; they too, have saved my life.
I just thank You Lord for everything, the list is long and mounting;
Many, many blessings ring and many more for counting!

And thank you God for Your dear Son, Jesus is His name,
He died to free us all from sin and did so without shame!
I'm thankful now for all the goals that Jesus had in mind;
The inspiration in His role was mighty and sublime,
For He is our foundation that everybody needs,
We sing in adoration for all His wondrous deeds.
I thank you Lord at all cost, I do without delay,
For You are there when I am lost, You meet my needs each day.

And last, not least, I thank you for a very precious prize;
The special one you gave me, a chance to be alive,
To see the morning sunrise, and know that I've survived!

❖❖❖❖❖

TIME LINE

I know I've lived a life of woe,
Called "running through the mill"
To feed a fire of lust desire,
My restless heart to fill,
And in that task I came to ask
If God would love me still...

Because I walked a sinners way,
Which trail was long and clear;
And every step I took each day
Brought my dear Jesus near,

For He alone my sins atone,
And this I so revere.
The path of life just goes so far,
My steps have dwindled few;
Where, there at last His hands I'll clasp,
My Lord is waiting true!

❖❖❖❖❖

GOD IS WATCHING US

God is watching us from heaven's way He sees us each and all;
In every way of come what may, He's there to catch our fall!
To tread a straight and righteous path, it should behoove us all;
To fear God's wrath, a mighty craft, but heed His loving call.

God is watching while we're sleeping too, and watches when we rise.
He's true to comfort weeping through, should lives go in demise.
He's by us when we're on the Job to keep us safe and warm,
Depend on God where dangers trod, to shelter us from harm.

He's light that takes the darkness out, adds hope for all despaired;
Calms doubts in all with starkness bouts of many folks despaired.
God is watching us and counting names, and keeping records too;
His very aims are staking claims, for those who make it through.

So, lift your eyes to God on high, return his lasting care;
And by and by you'll see Him nigh, amid the trumpets blare;
But cast your sight down to the ground; and shun your God above,
The devils pound will drag you down to Satan's flaming cove!

MY PILOT

In daily grind sometimes I find an urge to steal away,
To some lone spot, a peaceful lot, when I am in dismay,
So off I trot to that quiet spot, a forest stream or creek,
Where nature dines and beauty shines is company that I seek!

Where wild life croons their gleeful tunes in their own paradise...
God's scheme of things which clearly brings the wonders he applies.
Now resting here I sense Him near, His presence fills the air;
He's in the trees, He's in the leaves, the stream, He's everywhere!

Amidst the creek I hear Him speak in voice of rippling waves;
He's there in sight as geese take flight, a scene that memory saves.
While there I gaze through evening's haze in show of sunset's glow.
I see the leaves from trees fall free and drift on with the flow.

I see God's plan in thoughts I scan that man is like those leaves.
Who lives and dies before God's eyes in life that God so weaves,
Then on some river just drift forever in beauty of nature's realm.
Where one can say "No more dismay" with God there at the helm!

❖❖❖❖❖

WHY ?

Why is "why" the question? Here are my reasons why:
'Cause folks have no conception, which of course they may deny,
Some ask why of everything they do not understand,
And after someone answering, ask why one was so bland!

But why is not important, it's the answer that counts.
So please don't be so scant when giving the accounts.
Here are questions people ask, my list is just a few;
To understand this simple task, is think of it as true!

Why is the sky so often blue with all it's brilliant hue?
Because the clouds are none or few showing the color through?
Why does the mighty ocean roar like lions in their den?
Is it Neptune on the ocean floor beating his wife again?

Why is the earth so very round, when it looks to be so flat?
Was it because Columbus found a course upon his map?
You can ask why to everything, even ask why to why;
No simple answer does it bring, some folks don't even try.

Why is there anything? The answer lies above;
By hands of God, our only King, and by His trust and love.
Why no answer to anything? Only God knows reasons why.
All I know, His mercies bring the truth which we rely,
And my question is not why!

❖❖❖❖❖

HOW FIRM A FOUNDATION

Take any building structure in range from short to tall,
And having many sizes from huge to very small.
They all have one thing common, a low foundation wall.
Although it may look solid some weakness may exist;
Brought on by many factors that arises in its midst,
And as you view that building you may not see it list.

So as you look upon it, it may not be as well
As the sight that you are seeing, since you could never tell
That in this mighty body, weak foundations dwell.
Thus, the building is no stronger than the blocks it's resting on,
And the footing is no greater than the ground that spreads beyond.
With a weak foundation never does a body stand alone!

Now man is like that structure made by God on high,
His footing may have weakness but nothings looks awry.
His body's strong appearance deceives the human eye.
Thus, man is no more stronger than belief he's resting on,
And his steps are no more truer than the ground he treads upon.
And his footing is no surer than his will to overcome.

"How firm is your foundation? Does your standing list or sway?
Are your footsteps planted squarely upon this earthly clay?
Do you stand on your convictions? Are you solid when you pray?"
If you, your body's structure, meets this building code;
Then all the strength it musters never will erode!
Then all your life's endeavors can carry the heavy load.

So when your time has passed and you've met its every test;
You've strengthened every column where upon your structures rest,
You have met your builder maker you have done your very best!

❖❖❖❖❖

RIGHT DIRECTION

I surrender, I surrender. I've fought the battle long;
my life's been through a blender, it's time to right a wrong!
I surrender all my worry in my bosom held so tight!
I need to cease my hurry and slow down in my plight.

I surrender all my trophies that I have held so high;
and now my aim and hope is to bid them all good bye,
'cause I'm giving in to yearning, for much a better way;
my heart is ever burning for my place on judgment day.

I surrender my behavior, I'm climbing out the pits.
I'm turning to my savior, "I'm cashing in my chips!"
I'm turning down the thermostat, I'm pulling up my stakes;
I'm putting down the welcome mat for good of goodness sakes.

I surrender, I surrender, I shout it out today!
In joy I'm going in splendor, I go no other way.
I'm giving up, I'm quitting, "I'm throwing in the towel",
it's only quite befitting 'cause of the life I've fouled.

I surrender, 'cause I know it's wise; I'm calling it a day;
I'm locking up in paradise then throw the key away.
I'm traveling on my journey; I'm carrying no back pack;
I'm in a different tourney and I'm never looking back!

❖❖❖❖❖

AWAKENING

I was restless in my sleep last night, but waking up this morn,
I realize how nice and bright a new day will adorn.
I see the shadows on my wall from tree limbs in their sway.
Brings back the memories I recall in times of yesterday.

Those reflections now remind me of good times gone before,
And all my days that's left to be I'll cherish evermore.
Now I confess life's been a test with often "bumps to grind,"
But I intend to do my best whatever ways I find;

For in the past sometimes was cast a dose of life's hard sham;
But just like water from a glass, 'tis water o'er the dam;
So I must greet each coming day with good outlook on life,
By thinking in a faithful way, and not about the strife.

So now each morn when I awake, come either rain or shine,
I plan to rise and place my stake in all that's good and fine.
To meet the goals that I will set to carry on my way--
To stay the course without regret, and look to each new day!

LIFE'S CONTESTANTS

Life is merely a contest where simple rules apply,
And all participants entered will need to qualify,
In living by certain standards that's judged from heaven's eye.

The rules are really easy, but many to comprehend.
A test of right to follow with might where no rule shall suspend.
It's a test of will endurance in which everyone can win!

In this game of life competing and with its rule comply;
By joining with all contestants is ended with a tie,
Then all the first place honors are awarded by God on High!

❖❖❖❖❖

A VAGABOND'S DREAM

Over life's rushing river, down through the currents go;
Like a piece of old dead driftwood upon the tides I flow
To a better land I'm dreaming, where greener grasses grow.
The route may be rocky for this old loner be;
But my will is not to waver as these waters carry me--
To that peaceful spot I'm pining that lies beyond the sea.

'Cause I dream of peace and basking in grace and harmony.
Of faith and love that's lasting for all humanity,
But in this world existing, is little of this I see!
So I care not where this river takes me with chains that bond,
And when my journey's over with all my shackles gone,
I will rest in my blue heaven out in the vast beyond.
It will then be something greater for this lonely vagabond.

❖❖❖❖❖

CHARACTER

If within our lives there's heartache and pain or discomfort from sad despair,
We can alter this course by hope attain a solution to this affair.
With eyes, though weary, be restful and sure to look through strife we see;
With out thoughts less dull, our actions more pure, will bring us tranquillity.

If while in this task our conscience is clear in all the work we do;
And having the faith that we hold dear will see all of these projects through.
By spreading all of kindness galore, our woes will ever be few.
With all the joy and forgiveness in store will be changing our lives anew.

When showing respect for each and all, there's no better way it seems,
Being honest up front and standing tall are ever our ways and means.
Yes, we all must continue to live with hope, the highest of all supremes.
All these good traits will build up our scope and also our self esteems.

By placing trust in our Father above and also in everyone,
And giving to all our care and love will give us our strength to come.
When we add the traits of courtesy will upon our characters build.
And using good humor, we should agree, will contribute to all good will,
When these facts above, that lead to repent, are within our lives instilled,
And when our lasting days are spent, our goals have been fulfilled!

❖❖❖❖❖

LIVE IT UP

Both women and men are prone to sin, some do it intentionally.
If you're someone who meets this trend, consider this tip from me;
That when you sin don't sin so small, think big is how you view it;
'Cause on the way you'll surely fall with either way you do it.
And when you're lying tell 'em big! The small ones never mind;
For the largest deepest hole you dig is same for either kind;
And when you steal, don't waste your time by taking just small things;
Set your sights for larger find, either one, jail time brings!

When you're cheating don't settle for less, for cost will be the same;
'Cause while you're losing your nobleness, you also mar your name.
So as you live just live it big whatever your reasons be;
'Cause in the end you can't renege on your life's misery.
And yet, there is another way you can live your life more tall,
And that is brighten up every day attempting no sin at all!
By smiling when a frown is due or looking into some eyes,
And telling tales that's only true and not a pack of lies.

Letting tear drops fall in humble care with not a sole pretense,
Avoiding the pit falls of despair, a way that now relents.
Instead of stealing, do peace mealing with friends and foes alike.
helping people with good feeling, makes a rewarding strike!
And don't betray your fellow man, you'll need his help someday.
Reach out to him with willing hand, this bond will work its way.
So as you live, just live it big with these your choices be;
'Cause in the end...you won't renege on your morality!

THE HELPING STAND

I have seen along the road some sort of vegetable stand,
Where farmers towed their garden load to sell for what they can.
I met a man who has a stand, but sells no crops doe he.
What he has is help for man, and everything goes for free!
Above the door of his lil' store, a sign, The Helping Stand;
"I give assist with my own gifts, I give a helping hand."
When I went in to speak with him, no humbler man seemed bred.
With heavy sighs and tearful eyes this is what he said:
"I have much wealth from life of stealth, which is a well known fact,
But now my aim is cure the pain by giving it all back!
For in my life there's been much strife, I stepped on many toes,
So help me God on all I've trod, I'll end some others woes.
You wouldn't think a man would sink to rob poor people blind;
But down I sank to the lowest rank, and found no peace of mind.
Now I'm alone and need atone, I wish to set things right,
By giving back to those who lack, is now my guiding light.
Still, lone souls somewhere out there could use a helping hand,
So I'll show care for those despaired, if they'll visit my helping stand,
In my heart, in stages, a battle rages to square with all my sin.
I treated folks like mice in cages, it's now time to amend.
But there's a hitch in every stitch, with you it may save nine,
If in this cause you truly pitch to spread this wealth of mine.
You must not run, shun or hide when sharing with others my wealth,
What you receive, let your conscience lead... for all must need the help.
So now receive, and when you leave, go share these gifts I give,
Especially those in pain or bereaved, so they may happily live!
Then you will find at the end of your line, you missed the pitfall's stinging,
Then like me you'll forever be free as we join the angels singing!"

❖❖❖❖❖

ACTIVE MEMBER

I'd like to think as time goes by
that I'm the lucky one;
that I received my "piece of pie"
and my "place in the sun";
that I stood tall and met my call
and lived life's full demand;
by doing right to each and all
with trust and helping hand;

that I was there in their despair
to comfort or console,
and ease the pain they came to bear
when miseries unfold.
Now I'm no saint nor preacher man,
but have my own desires,
to have a will to build good will,
to do what God inspires,

and I believe I pay my dues
for life's both joy and woe.
Each day I live I try to choose
the best ways that I know,
but in our chain of life we
find a missing link or two;
it may have been some fault of me,
or maybe some by you,
but either way I'm bound to try,
to dedicate my best,
to do what's right by God on high,
and He will do the rest!

BEST CHOICE

We wake up every morning
and we go to bed each night.
We spend each day performing
a thing that's wrong or right,
but do we ever stop to think
just what our choices are?
Do we ever reach a final brink
of having gone too far?

Do we ever realize a better way to go?
To do the things that satisfies
to give our lives more glow!
There are two choices in our life,
the first, the best I know;
is holding on to Jesus Christ,
the next, is let Him go;
but I suggest you cling to Him,
as He upon the cross,
bearing all the brunt of sin
and did so with remorse,

but if you choose to let him
go your life will always be;
an empty thing that struggles
so and ends in misery,
but take the Lord within your breast,
accept Him as your own,
your very soul will come to rest
with Jesus at the throne!

❖❖❖❖❖

THE STRANGER

The rain drops poured and thunder roared as lightning winked its eye,
and from a bolt, a crashing jolt came surging from the sky!
I crouched into the last row pew in our small country church,
and through the back way I could view a scene my eyes would search.
For storm winds pried the door aside, I peered out in the maze;
and found myself just mystified at frightening lightning rays.
A crashing sound came all around and echoed on the soar,
and through and through it shook each pew and rumbled with its roar.
The congregation hushed their song, the great "Amazing Grace",
when vibrants strong that came along just shook that holy place...
...and from the night and flashing light, and from the rain's downpour,
there came a sight mid thunder's might, a man stood at the door!
A thinly man quite wan and bland with headband and a beard,
his clothes were worn and tattered torn, a sight that just appeared!
'Tis a vagabond someone said: "Just homeless on his way,
out looking for a place to spread and for the night to stay",

but in he came from torrent rain caught everybody's eye!
For clothes he wore from core to core, was dry as dry is dry...
...and there behold on door's threshold stood he who looked half dead;
...a contrast pales to mighty gales that raged on overhead;
and suddenly there was no sound which silence stole away...
...'twas just as loud as any cloud that burst a lightning ray.
Then all eyes scanned the lonely man who strolled down through the
aisle.
His speech began at the pulpit stand, a sermon heard a mile.
So, he preached on with a mighty tone that held us in his spell,
a total stranger in our midst, declaring war on hell!
He knew the Bible front to back and not once did he look...
he did not lack nor was he slack on words from that good book.
He preached away and I must say: "I never saw the sort",
this stranger man at the pulpit stand just flowing with rapport.
Then, all around came thunder down and lightning struck its mark,
and overhead the lights went dead and left us in the dark...
but, in due time the lights were fine but, folks don't comprehend,
for at the stand the bearded man had disappeared within.

So, who was he, this mystery, will he ever show anon?
Was he a man with blood that ran? Was he a mere icon?
The Holy One, God's truly Son who put us to the test?
Or just a bum who's "on the rum", I guess we only guess!

❖❖❖❖❖

ONLY THE LONELY

There are concrete prisons in each state where real crooks do their time,
but other cells where lonely dwells are ones in "state of mind!"
For those are prisons in some lives without the walls or bars.
They strangle-hold the lonely souls who's coping with their scars.
Some have sentences up to life with no parole in sight,
and they will stay in their dismay as victims in their plight.

When, who, or where, come judges' care? Have they no heart or soul?
Compassionless and emptiness, too oblivious to console!
It is a world where pains unfurl in someone's comfort search;
and bitter ends may find no friends, just others who besmirch.
It's a sad, sad thing when some hearts sting when pierced by a poisonous word,
but worst of all is to hear no call with only silence heard.

And the lonely cell is a life of hell in jail without a gate;
but the prisoners there have a common share, they sit alone and wait.
Wait by the way-side lest they find some inner self release,
to live with fain, and not by pain for everlasting peace.
Peace! Ah peace! What a gracious thing in a world where folks need love,
where they live on and be unknown, except to God above.

And someday comes for the lonesome ones when peace will come to all,
for heaven waits for the lone inmates, who receive their only call!

❖❖❖❖❖

IT TAKES ONLY ONE BLESSING

When evening shadows come to fall
at close of weary days,
count your many blessings all,
not sorrows or dismays,

for oftentimes we dwell on woes,
and often we forget;
that even though ill winds may blow,
means not our end is met,

for God has given us a gift,
our lives, for which we owe;
to Him our very soul we lift
when hard times come to tow,

and every blessing that we count
dispels so many ills,
and conquer mountains we surmount
with strength which God instills.

THE MASTER PLAN

God has a plan that never fails,
it's one that guides us all,
through many times of dreary spells
and lifts us should we fall;

and fall we will if footsteps tread
down life's lone rocky trail;
forgetting how Christ's blood was shed
and pain that He befell...

Forgetting that He braved the cross
to save our souls from hell...
seeing His cause as just a loss
and not our Father's will...
but in the Master's scheme of things
He wants the world to see:
that Jesus Christ, the King of Kings,
is hope for you and me...

That we must act upon His plan
by every sin confess,
and bonding with out fellow man
to bring us happiness.

By holding trust and care in Him
to glorify His name...
and show compassion to all men
will satisfy His aim...

and last, not least, is loyalty
with will to understand:
that having faith in God's decree...
will guarantee His plan!

❖❖❖❖❖

MASTER ARTIST

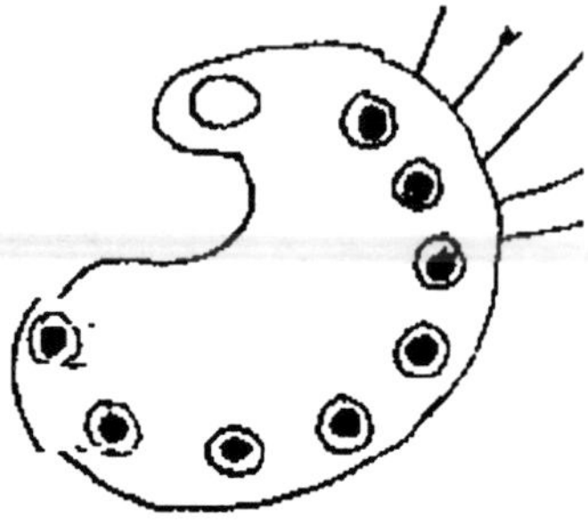

There is a master artist
From a far away land
Who painted the mountains
And the canyons grand.

He colored the crimson
In the sunset's glow,
Then finished the highlights
On a great rainbow!

He mixed up purple
For the morning dawn,
VanDyke brown
For the yearling fawn.

He painted the greens
In the whispering pines,
Then did their needles
With His pure fine lines.

He sketched in the oceans
That run so deep,
Then painted them with motions
That forever keep.

He brushed in the shadows
In the river's flow,
And painted the fields
Where the flowers grow.

He painted the sky
With His brilliant blue,
Then put in the clouds
With their silver hue,

And then in black
Came the dark midnight,
But also the shine
Of the bright moon light.

Then there's Jupiter,
Pluto, and mars,
And He rounded out the Universe
With twinkling stars.

Now His masterpiece is finished
With a wonderful glow,
And the artist smiles from Heaven,
His studio!

❖❖❖❖❖❖❖❖

THE MASTER ARCHITECT

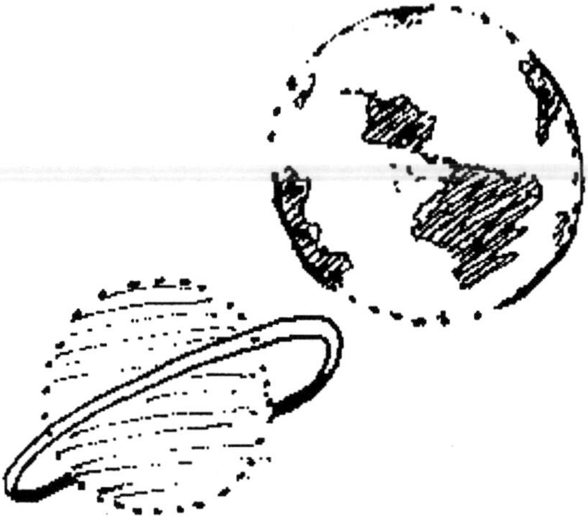

He is the master architect
Who surveyed all the world.
With wonders grand He drew a plan
For creation to unfurl.

He formed the world with powers great
And after this was done;
He built the skies for light to rise,
For this, He made the sun.

And in the beauty of the night
His wonders now unveil
The full moon bright with silver light
And stars that cast their spell!

His splendid touch of master's art
Brought forth the mighty earth,
He then proceeds to sow the seeds
That gave all natures birth.

And as the master architect,
He structured each and all,
With greatest ease He formed the seas,
And carved the mountains tall.

He planted all the woodlands free
With dear and loving things;
And it is here that we can hear
The songs that nature sings.

He cut away the earthly clay
To meet the river's flow,
And filled these streams with sunlit gleams
To make these waters glow!

He is the greatest architect,
And this His greatest dream;
To complete His plan, creating man,
And finish up His scheme.

But left in store was one last chore
And this will so be done.
To give to us the one we trust,
Lord, Jesus Christ, His Son!

HEART OPERATION

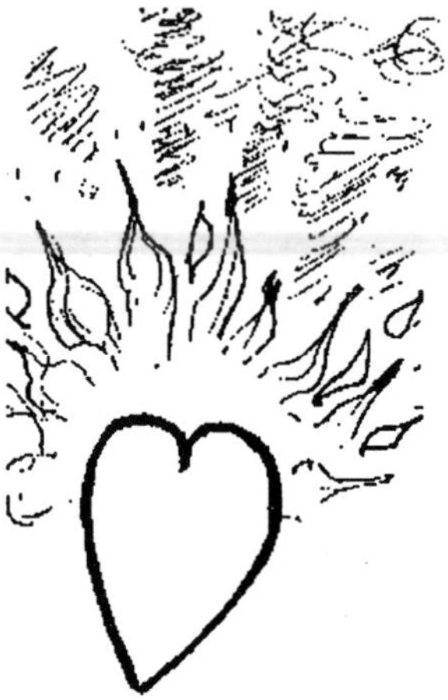

My heart was operated on
To undergo repair;
The surgeon was the best, bar
none,
Or I would not have fared.

For many years I felt the pain
And did not seek His hand,
And many times I wept in vain,
Just hid away or ran!

Until the day the moment came
My troubles reached a peak,
For in my heart had come a flame,
And help I went to seek.

I felt the need then to appeal
To one I trust the most;
I knew my heart would have to heal
Or everything was lost!

So in my plight my fear took flight,
I bade the surgeon in.
He made it all come out alright,
For I feel great again!

I now can tread with head up high
And proudly I can trod,
Because the surgeon I relied
'Twas my almighty God!

THE MAN UPSTAIRS

With hopes and cares for "The Man Upstairs"
I search for His guiding light;
I yearn for His will for my heart to fill,
For a need in my earthly plight!

I have no gold, but I have a soul
Which is wealth of my whole affairs!
It's the gift He gave, it's the one He saved
By the grace of "The Man Upstairs".

And "The Man Upstairs" with our soul He spares
If we follow His Master plan,
Is believe in Him and confess our sin,
And be kind to our fellow man!

And look to Him when our lives grow dim,
To His wonders that never cease,
And when in doubt throw the devil out,
Assuring us lasting peace.

Now the days go by and my time draws nigh,
Nothing that I see compares;
To the blessed love and the cares above,
Coming from "The Man Upstairs".

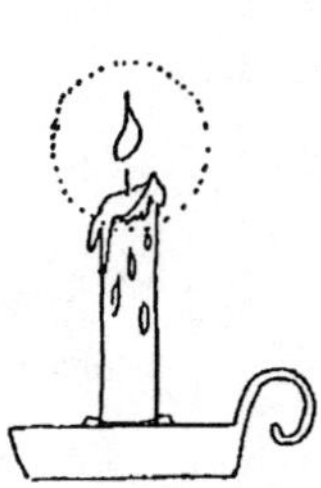

❖❖❖❖❖❖❖❖❖❖

MY PLEA

Oh Lord, can't I have one small amount
Of those precious blessings that I count?
For I've tried hard, I've stood the test.
I always did what you deemed best.
Now it's time to sum it up
And see how high I filled my cup.
And now in my humble way,
Searching for peace with every day,
I pray to Thee with anxious heart
With all my sins to Thee impart.

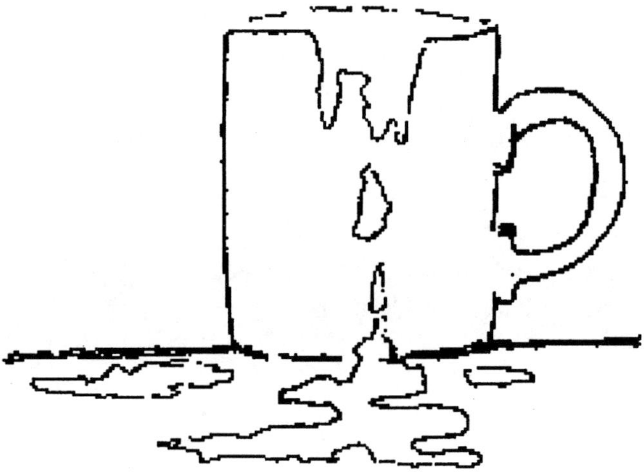

❖❖❖❖❖❖❖❖❖

IT'S ONLY TEMPORARY

Beyond those darkest clouds we see
That hover oft' on high,
Are better things for you and me
That cometh by and by!

No matter how much gloom we feel
Or ills we have to bear;
We always gain our strength and will,
And hope, that's found in prayer.

So all together let us pray
To God, with voice as one;
And all dark clouds will fade away,
And leave us in the sun.

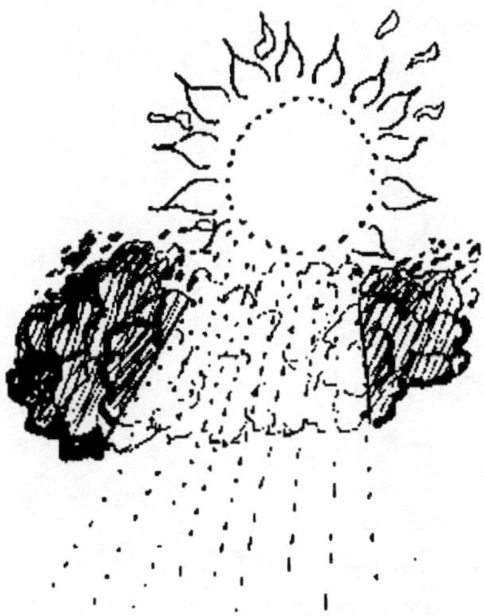

7 DAYS WITHOUT GOD MAKES ONE WEAK!

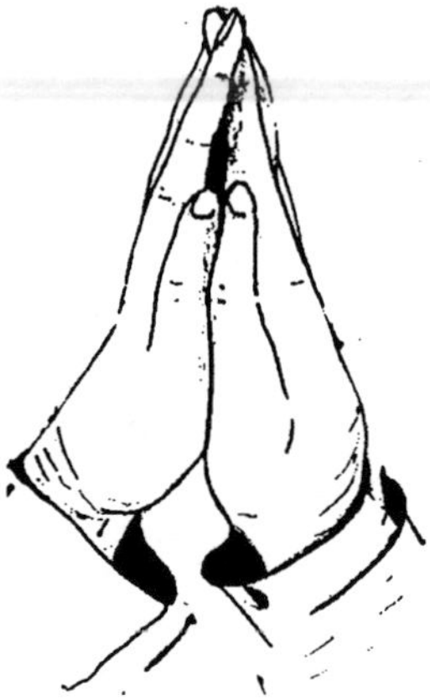

Do you feel down trodden
And sad with emptiness?
Or that you've been forgotten
And your life is in a mess?
And your mind is so annoyed
That this has made you weak?
And you need to fill this void,
But you have no clues to seek?

For these questions I'm
proposing,
There's something you can do.
It will lead you to eroding
The ills affecting you!

The answer is to follow
With a very strong belief,
Every day that's hollow
With a will to deal with grief.

Just start each day with Monday
And pray with all your might,
And when you reach next Sunday,
Your goal should be in sight!

For on that day--surrender
Every ill that you possess,
And God is there so tender
To take them from your breast.

DAILY REMINDER

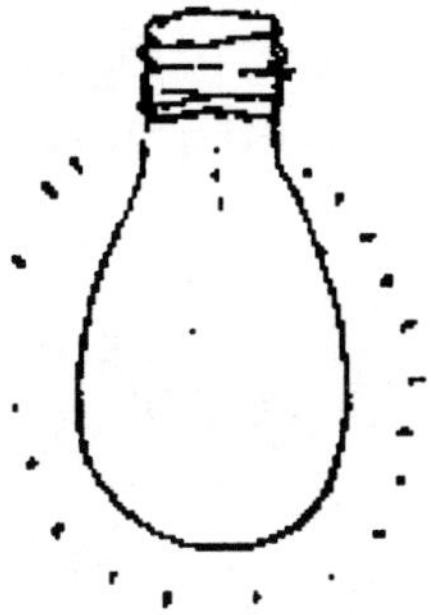

Comes often times when quietness
finds
Me in a pensive mood;
I hear a sound that's so profound,
It brings me solitude.

The sound I hear is sweet and free,
A voice so soft and clear;
Calling, calling, calling me
To bring me closer near.

It is the voice of Christ I hear,
I hear Him with my heart;
He takes away my woes and fear
And gives my life new start.

He fills my cup, He lifts me up,
And talks to me each day;
He's here abrupt to interrupt
The ills that come my way!

❖❖❖❖❖❖❖❖

RIVER OF LIFE

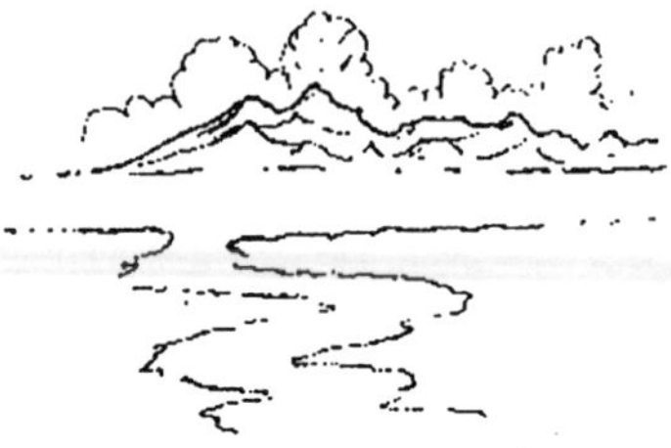

Over the river of life we flow,
Down the currents we sail,
Upon the changing tides we go
Fighting it tooth and nail!

It is a long and rocky route
For all us sailors be;
But many will reach their goals
throughout
Or sink within the sea.

We're traveling with a hope for peace,
Of love and harmony;
And striving for our wars to cease--
'Til everyone is free.

So we're sailing on this river of life
To some far better place,
Where absent are the woes and strife,
Where life is not a waste.

❖❖❖❖❖❖❖❖

KNOCK, KNOCK, WHO'S THERE?

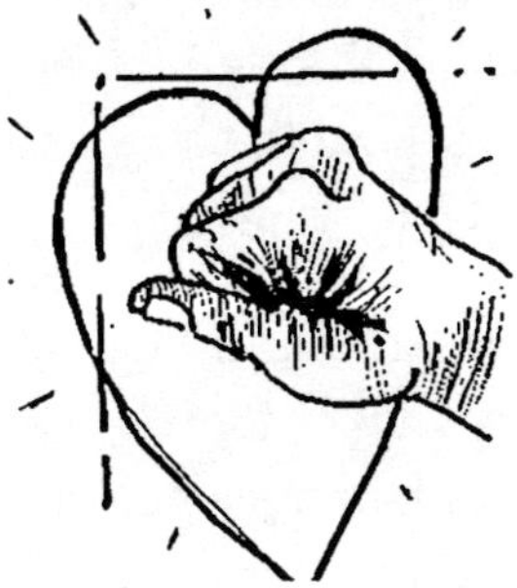

Who on my heart strings is
knocking?
The door is open you see.
Long has my misery been
locking
And churning inside of me.

Who in my heart now is
pounding?
And sending it up to soar,
This feeling of joy surrounding
My heart as never before!

Who from my heart now has captured
My sin, my loneliness and hate?
And sparing my soul to be raptured
Cometh the judgment date.

Who in my life now has saved me
From pits of despair, discord?
Who lifts me so sublimely?
'Tis Jesus Christ my Lord!

HEAVEN'S ENTRY

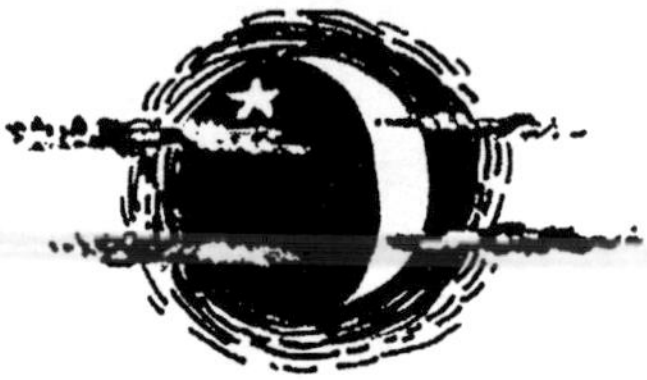

There is a magical stairwell
That spirals up through the sky;
It winds up where the angels dwell
To mighty God on high!

It is my hope to climb that way
To meet my maker there,
To be within His presence stay
And gain eternal care.

The trail is rocky I surmise
But I will carry on
Until I reach my paradise,
My cverlasting home!

Where God upon the throne He rests
With Jesus by His side,
Where I'll receive eternal bliss
By trusting and abide.

❖❖❖❖❖❖❖❖

BEYOND THE SEA

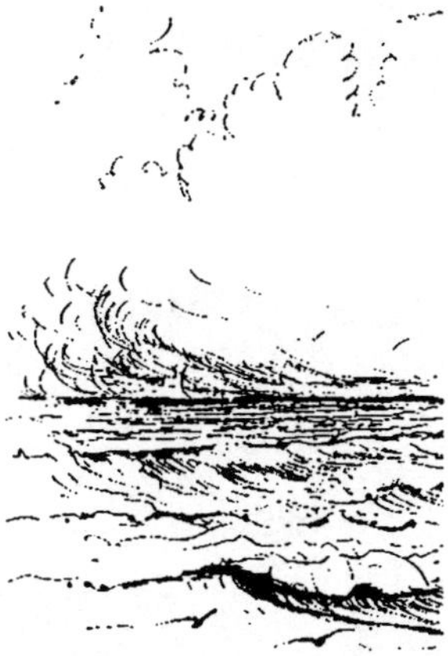

Upon my lofty perch I view
Across the mystic sea,
A stretch of never ending blue
That spreads on endlessly.

It climbs up to the spacious
skies
On into Heaven's Gate,
And winds its way through
Paradise
Where God and angels wait.

Beyond horizon's secret
realms
My yearning heart explores,
Like captains at their guiding helms,
In search for safer shores.

Somewhere beyond the rolling waves
This gateway beckons me;
And in my soul a calmness stays,
While searching to be free!

HOME AT LAST

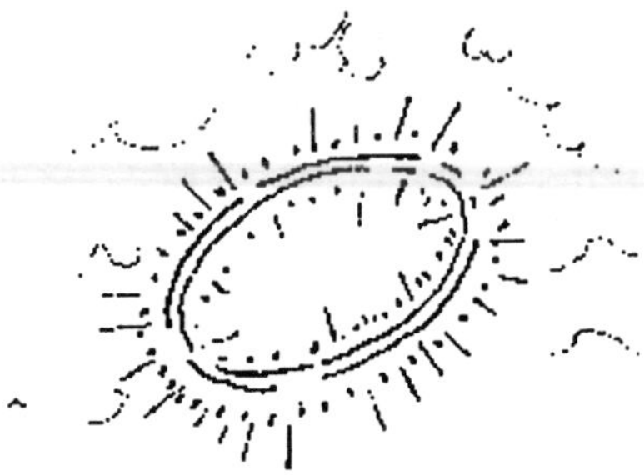

I know it's true
Without ado,
From heaven God will
call;
If I believe and I concede
That Jesus died for all!

God will forgive
When I re-live
And ask in Jesus' name;
For it was He who set me
free,
And thus my glory came!
So now I'm blessed,
My sins confessed,
Assures my entry there;
Through heaven's door, forevermore,
With all God's love to share.

❖❖❖❖❖❖❖❖

THE ONLY COURSE

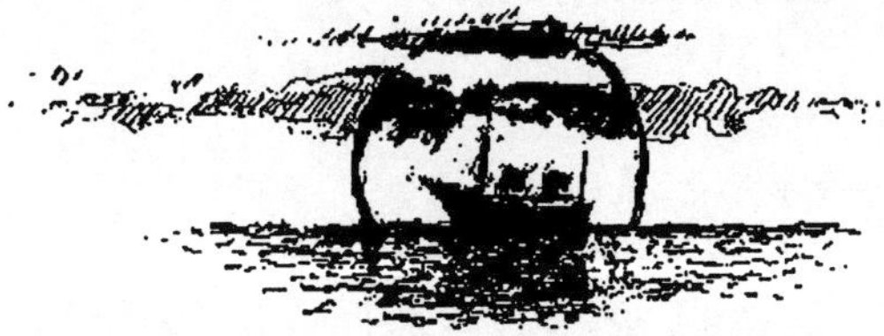

You do not need an aeroplane
Or rocket made of late,
To reach an altitude to gain
Your way to heaven's gate.

All you need is love and prayer
And hopeful sacrifice,
By showing all respect and care
In the name of Jesus Christ.

For if the love you have for Him
Is shown to one and all,
Your guiding light will never dim
And you will never fall!

So when you pray and show remorse
And receive God's son today,
That's charting out your only course
On God's heavenly way!.

❖❖❖❖❖❖❖❖

LIGHT THE WAY

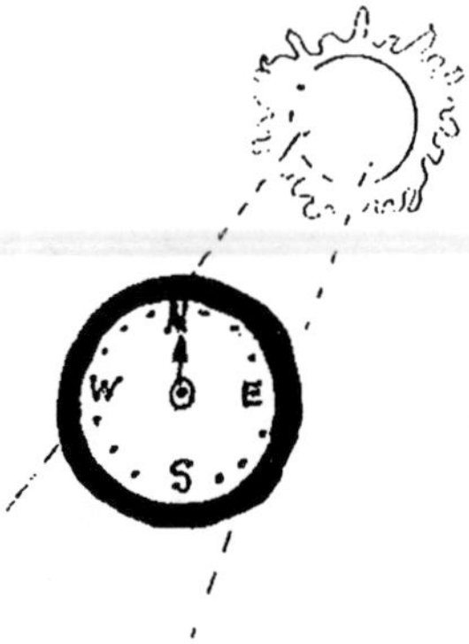

Dear Lord, please come to me
today
And bear my troubles here,
Somewhere enroute I've lost my
way,
I need a course to steer.

The path I'm on is dimly lit,
I hardly see it clear.
I'm treading on it bit by bit
To ease away my fear.

I know your light is what I need
To brighten up the route,
For every rock that I impede
I need to sort it out.

I need you now most urgently
To set my compass straight,
So I can handle all I see,
For time is getting late!

❖❖❖❖❖❖❖❖❖

SOMETIME

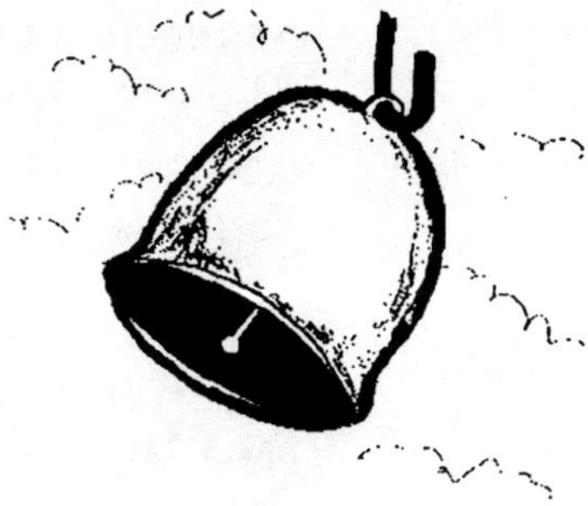

I stand upon the edge of time,
The distant drums I hear.
The tolling of the bells that
chime
Brings me solace here.

I look on high with anxious
eye
To search the sky above;
I see God's presence coming
nigh,
I feel His warmth and love.

The magic of this moment brings
A joy I've never known,
For soon I'll see the King of Kings
Who is my very own.

OPEN UP

Surrender all your lives to God,
Allow His spirit in.
And every path you choose to trod
Forgives you for your sin.

Let Jesus be a friend indeed,
Dear Christ, His only Son.
He'll satisfy your every need
From now to Kingdom come.

So open up your minds and hearts
To His everlasting care,
And all the blessings He imparts,
When you talk to Him in prayer.

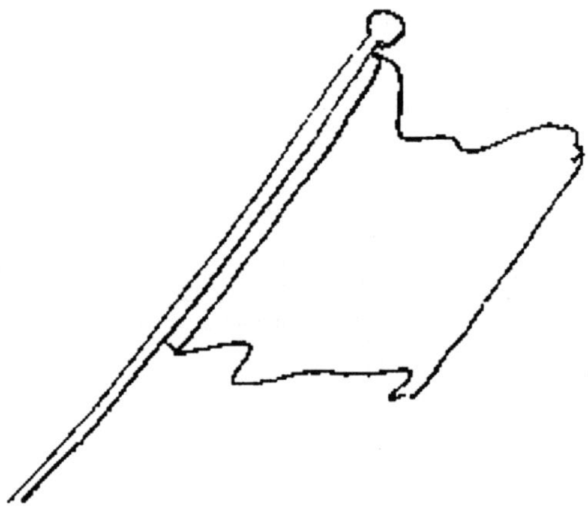

THE BOOK

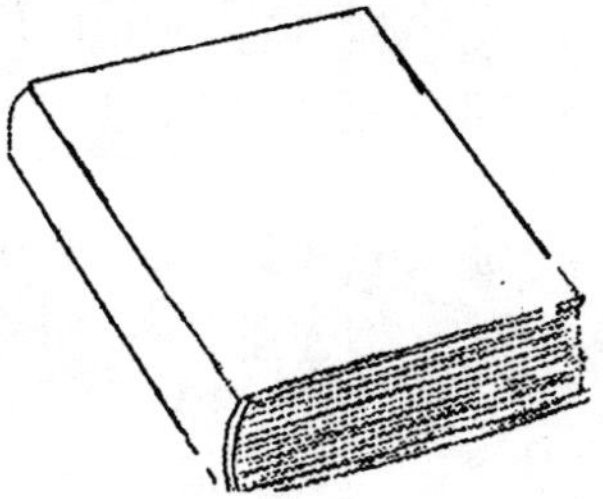

There is a great day coming soon,
I feel I cannot wait.
I hear the shrill of the bugler's tune,
The rapture of my fate.

I hear the drone of the drummer's
 sound,
An aurora seen on high.
I feel His presence so profound
As His judgment day draws nigh.

And He will come as He did before,
But this time in His hands;
He'll hold the names He has in store
In His great known Book of Lambs.

And listed there are special ones,
His goal, to set them free;
Their very soul for which He comes,
And one of them is me!

THE LOST LAMB

I bow my head in shame dear
Lord
For long neglecting Thee.
I have been living by the
sword,
But still, you stayed by me.

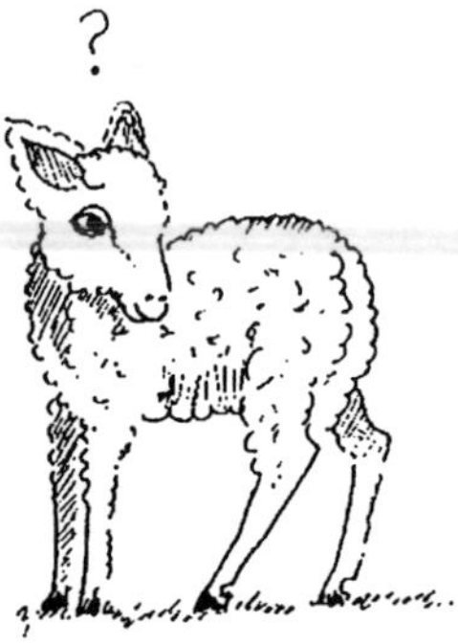

I knew that you were always
there
And yet I turned an eye,
And many times I felt despair
When you were there close by.

I looked for strength another way
Down life's deep darker lane,
And this poor lamb who went astray
Is now endowed with pain.

Please bring me back into the fold
Beneath your guiding hand.
Oh Lord, my life has been so cold,
I need your warmth again!

So now I bow my head and pray,
And humbly go to Thee;
To ask forgiveness for the way
I failed you miserably.

Now in my heart there's hope I feel
Your holy presence here,
And in my life a void will fill
As long as you are near.

HOMEWARD BOUND

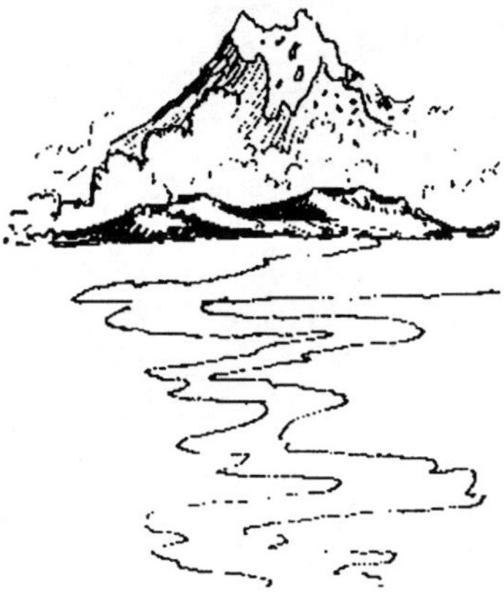

I'll sail this river wherever it goes,
I'll go where it takes me.
I'll follow this river of life that flows
With all its mystery.

I'll search for my Savior when following down
To that beautiful valley below.
I'll join with my Jesus where there He is found,
And He is waiting, I know.

I'll sail on this river, this river I'm on.
I'll follow these waters so free.
I know this journey will lead me home
To my heaven in glory be.

ENDURANCE

A vision that my mind has seen,
The cross where Jesus died;
He, stretched upon its hefty
beam
So painfully crucified!

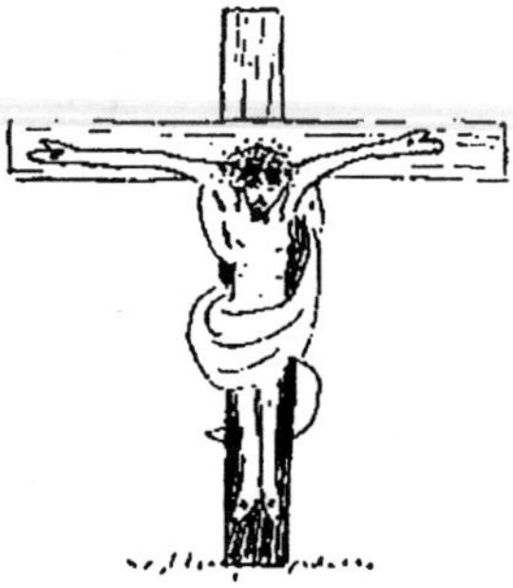

I vow myself to view Him there,
His body limp and pale
From all the pain He came to
bear
With every driven nail!

I set my sight on Calvary
Where once my Lord was slain,
If He suffered in this deed for
me,
Can't I endure my pain?

So when I feel my misery,
My thoughts go back to bear
The scene I see at Calvary,
And my Savior clinging there!

And all my troubles seem to fade
While peace fills up my heart;
For all the promises that He made
From my bosom never part.

MY SAVIOR LIVES WITHIN ME

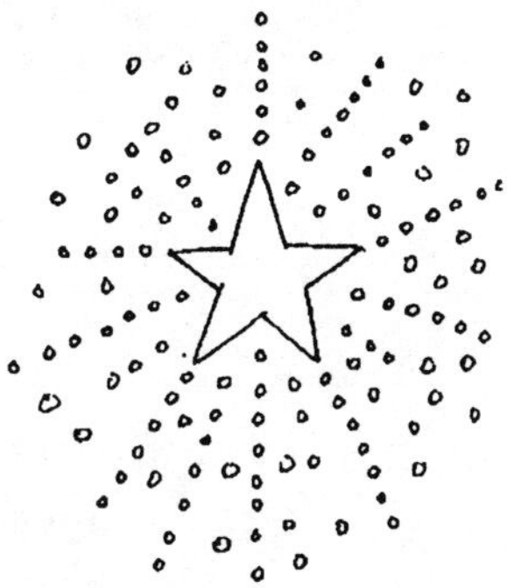

My Savior lives within my
life's
Pure sacred places dear;
I yearn for heaven's paradise
That brings me comfort
here.

I rise up when the morning
calls
With Jesus on my mind;
And when the evening dark-
ness falls,
He's made my day sublime!

Dear Jesus lives within my soul
And holds my spirits high,
And many thoughts of Him I hold
As time goes marching by.

And in my heart I'll hold Him there
From now to glory be;
Where all my troubles He will bear--
--Lasting Eternally.

IN HIS HANDS

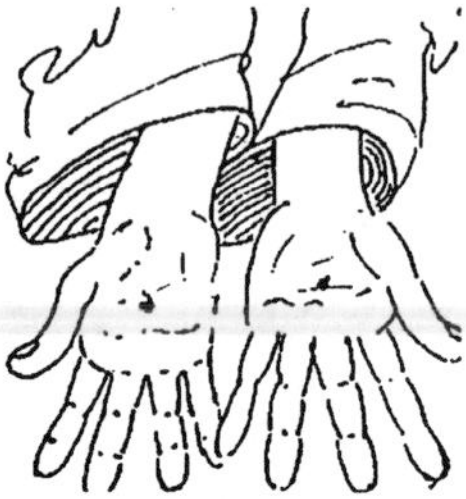

I hear the distant thunder roar,
I see the lighting sky,
I feel a spirit in me soar,
For God is drawing nigh!

I feel His storm within my veins.
I feel the rushing flow.
The very force in which He reigns,
That everyone should know!

The mighty wrath of God prevails
Within His powerful hands;
As raging winds of awesome gales
To those He reprimands.

But do not fear the storm, I say,
But God to whom you bow,
To fear Him, love Him, and obey,
Will bring the finest hour.

So through the storm its love to seek,
And not His hands of wrath;
For fearing God is not seen weak,
But strength in glory's path!

ONE CROSS FOR ALL

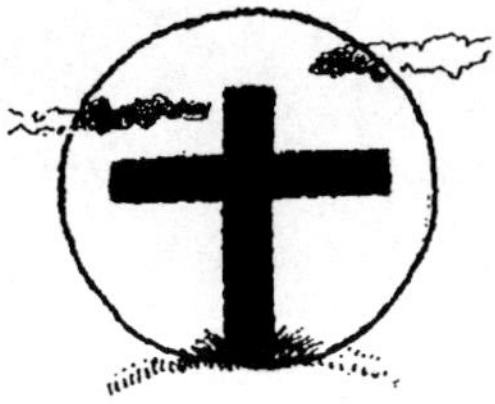

Have mercy Lord, Oh precious Lord,
I pray not just for me;
For other ones, whose hurting comes,
Are worse than mine can be.

No matter how I suffer here
With all my aches and pain;
Some others' ill is rougher still
On this old misery lane.

But it's a path we all will tread
To deal with vicious woe,
The many things that dreading brings,
That living has in stow.

For I've seen the smiling faces shine
Of those who walk with pain,
Of many found with braces bound,
And ones who live in vain.

The ones whose limbs are paralyzed,
The folks who cannot see,
Who offers me a token fee
By responding so happily!

And I feel my own ill dwindle down
As their courage reaches me.
For in my heart a flame they start
As they turn my thoughts to thee.

For you're the one who suffered most
Through all your love and care,
It's our remorse beneath the cross,
Of the pain you had to bear!

❖❖❖❖❖❖❖❖

OUR WAY

There's a need for inspiration, a daily revelation,
Something that will guide us on our way
To our destiny and love, to our heaven high above,
Where everyone will meet some sweet day.

And the hour is getting late, and many cannot wait
To meet their Mighty Maker in the sky;
Surely time will come as does the setting sun,
We will see our loving Savior by and by.

In all our future pain it will never be in vain,
For our Lord has taken care of that:
'Cause He suffered on the cross so there would be no loss,
So every single soul could adapt.

Now upon each precious hour do not hide nor cower,
Simply rectify to God and pray;
This is a good solution to relieve us of confusion
And clear the many objects in our way.

Because our goal is heaven, we count each day to seven,
On each, we have a duty to fulfill;
To love our God and neighbors, to stay in their good favors,
And to all endearing friends show good will.

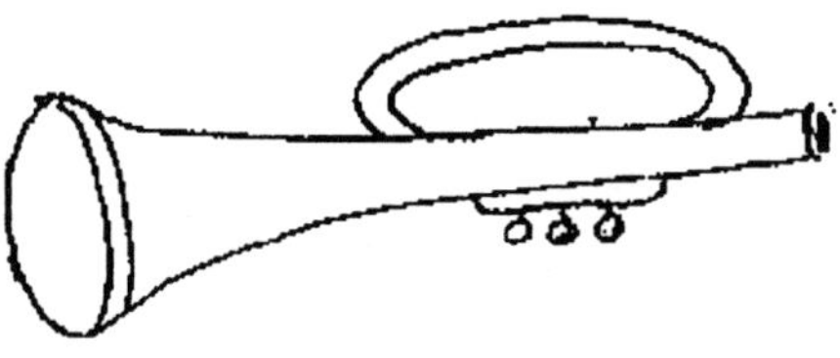

❖❖❖❖❖❖❖❖

A GREATER FORCE

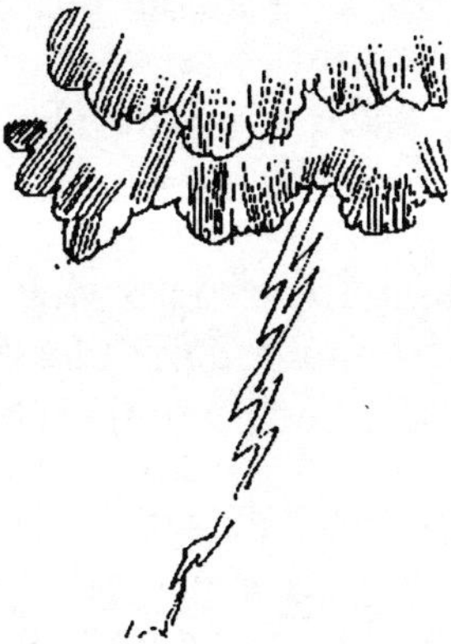

There is no power here on earth
 Can match the one above.
There is no force that's given birth
 Can win as much as love.

Of all the mighty guns of war
 None have gained a friend,
But all the care of friends that are,
 Brings strength that comes within.

It is the hand of God that rules
 In spite of what men say.
It is the greed that make men fools
 And leads them all astray.

And blood may flow along the way
 By some misguided deed,
And one may choose to live each day
 Without a care to heed.

But in the end he'll surely fall
 With all his thoughts to deem,
For when he comes to gain his pall,
 It's God, his judge supreme!

FLAME

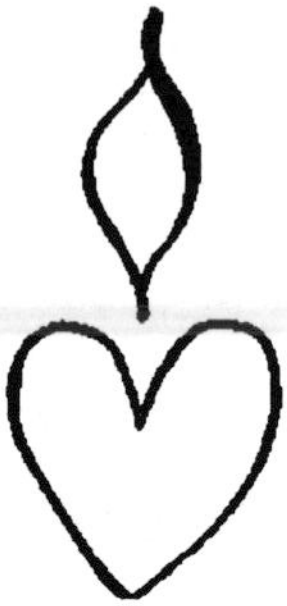

Lord, I have this passion burning
Down deep within my heart;
Stemming from years of yearning
And searching for where thou art.

I've lost my way a plenty
Along life's rocky way,
But I counted my blessings many
As I called on you each day.

And the road seems never ending
As I tread each careful step,
Avoiding the pitfalls pending,
Of which I'm not adept.

'Cause I had my times to falter
As I tried to do what's right,
And I strived in life to alter
Those wrongs I could not sight,

But this flame that I'm attending
I never want to douse;
Because I am depending
On the strength that you arouse.

And some day way up yonder
When the burning will decease,
I will never more need wonder,
For I will have my peace!

❖❖❖❖❖❖❖❖

THE JOURNEY FORWARD

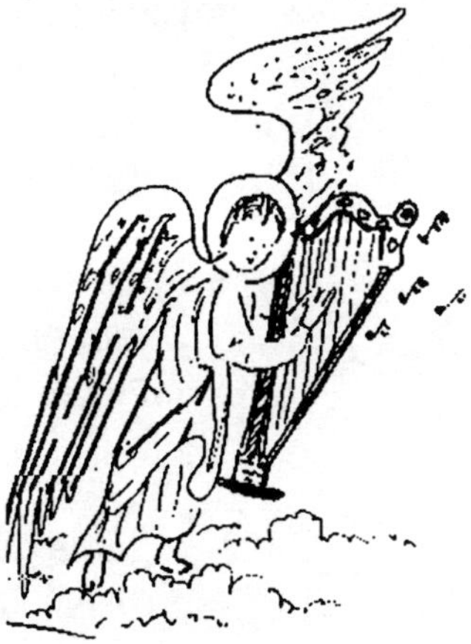

There's a paradise up yonder
Where I'm yearning for in
wonder,
Where I'll meet my precious
maker some sweet day;
For I know He's up there wait-
ing and has my hopes inflating,
As I find my inner peace along
the way.

For in this world I've wandered
And all its mysteries pondered,
And many times I've felt the
sting of pain;
Of a heart that has been riven, but God has so forgiven,
And I've learned to know His love is not in vain.

So from this world departing
I find it so rewarding,
As I sight my golden mansion way up there;
With the blaring trumpets blowing,
Where my lonely soul is going,
Where I hear the harps of angels everywhere!

Where my journey will complete
On a diamond studded street,
At last I'll reach my precious home;
Where Jesus, God reside, I will ever more confide,
And from then I know I'll never be alone.

THE BEST SIDE

Whatever we plot, wherever we prop,
Or whether we help it or not;
We're on a path of eternal wrath
If the strife in our life don't stop!

Some wallow each day in hollow dismay
And I wonder if they stop to pray?
If praying they don't, Its trouble they want,
And their problem will stay that way!

So to each his own whether young or grown,
Each one has his own life to hone;
And try they must to pry the lust
And evil from all who's prone.

Now there is a side all should take pride,
And that is to goodness subscribe.
And gain the strength and lose all the taint
That strives in our lives to thrive.

So let's all pitch in and cast away sin
And with a new life begin;
Where on judgment date at the pearly gate,
Our friend will lead us within.

"TURMOIL"

It's quite obvious turmoil in this country continues to prevail. The crime rate, teenage pregnancies, drugs, are the main culprits building at the heart of our problems. It's so sad and frustrating to have a cloud of violence dominating our news cast on every occasion without any relief in sight.

There are many reasons why these life styles by certain individuals have taken place, lack of jobs, divorced parents, and peer pressures are some of the suggested reasons, so what are the solutions?

I believe it lies with our leaders, the president, congress, and especially a change in our T.V. programming industry, and a better awareness among all of us, to do what we can on a local basis.

It would have far reaching effects across our country by coming together in our neighborhoods as a start.

The following 3 verses, "With Every Passing Day", "There Is No Justice", and "Daily Grind" are strictly my opinions as I have come to view and understand the situations in our land. They are not intended to offend anyone with my expressions within them.

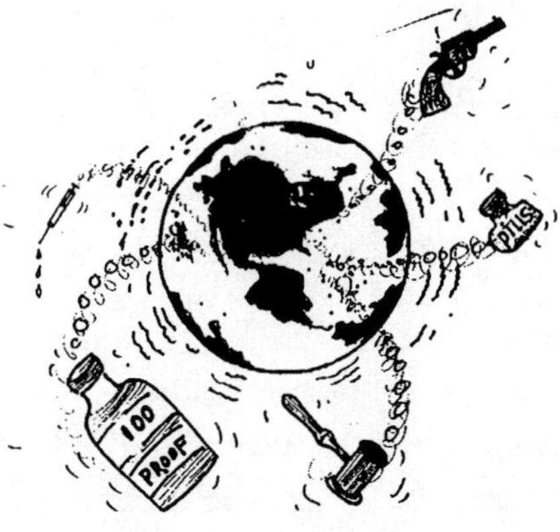

WITH EVERY PASSING DAY

I see two separate worlds
In our country, U.S.A.
On one side good will unfurls,
The other, in disarray.

I stand e.pluribus unum,
I'm here to state my say
Concerning the troubled portion
Living in disarray.

The evil side is tearing
The better side apart,
By forcing strife and fearing
To enter the people's heart.

Their image is wroth destruction,
Permissiveness, their trend.
Giving credence to corruption
Is to guarantee our end!

Within the years foregoing
I've seen this country slide
With its gusty ill winds blowing
As it brought us to divide.

We're in a deep depression,
Not one that banks may claim,
But a show of mass expression
That keeps coming from the brain!

'Cause it comes from years of failing
To properly live and think
About life styles prevailing,
Which is causing us to sink!

It's a chain-like noose that's winding
Around our necks to stay,
It continues 'round us binding
Now with every passing day!

The hour is nigh upon us,
We're 'bout to take a fall,
Unless they lose their greedy lust
That seems to strangle all.

Our nation now is crumbling
With all its moral decay.
Both drugs and crimes are rumbling
By some people gone astray.

Teenage girls in pregnancy,
Alarming is their count;
Inflating immorality
Toward an upward mount.

And disease is rampart running,
Creating much dismay.
The number of deaths are stunning
Here with every passing day!

There's hate, divorce, rejection,
And violence in the race;
And we've reached an intersection
At a cross roads we must face.

We were once an admiration
For all the world to see;
And once a great elation
Whence came the brave and free,

But is now a wide division
Expanded on our land,
By indulging in remission
Here is hard to understand!

What's happened in our nation
For strife to overwhelm?
Could it be an aberration
By our leaders at the helm?

'Twould be a great sensation
Within my heart and mind,
To win with acclamation
Back our streets just one more time.

Where we can go with much delight
And breathe the freedom air,
And safely walk the streets at night
Without the thoughts of fear!

The answer lies in striving
With all our will and might;
By removing those depriving
Us and educate what's right,

And mold us back again as one
And peace again to stay;
Enjoy the battle that we won
With every passing day!

THERE IS NO JUSTICE

Now I believe it's all naive
To think we're at our best.
Just look around, it can be found,
Corruption and unrest!

It's up to us to stop this fuss,
And try to put an end
To all the wrong that goes along
With this injustice trend.

For there is no justice in our land,
I'll list the reasons why:
The one main cause is in our laws
Which some folks don't rely.

We live each day in sheer dismay,
Some strive to do what's right,
But can't make gains without a change
By others in the plight.

We're caught up in a dreadful trend,
Permissiveness prevails,
Where lawyers spin to cover sin
To keep crooks out of jails.

The fault, it lies in judge's eyes,
In juries that are blind,
For when some creep kills in the street,
No verdict will they find!

But if they do they send them to
Some gorgeous jail motel.
They treat them nice like paradise,
Instead of prison's hell!

It is a shame they find no blame,
It sends a message strong,
That it's O.K. to rob and slay
And brush away their wrong.

The lawyers lie, the juries sigh,
And some of them will weep
Of some poor guy who goes awry,
And not his temper keep.

This same loco not long ago,
Who with a knife did slit
His young wife's throat, he came to gloat
When a wet eyed jury split,

'Cause of a tale he wept and wailed,
'Cause his Dad ran out on him,
When his Mama died, he felt denied
And his age was only ten.

Well, I say to you if this is true
Then we're all caught in harm's way,
'Cause all the folks who have these strokes
Will kill instead of pray!

Well, again he's back, this one eyed Jack,
Lying 'bout another kill.
And the judge, he blinks, the defense stinks,
And the jury winks,
And the system's lost its will!

And they'll do once more what they did
before,
And again this guy will walk,
And for fame he'll look and write a book,
And do TV and talk.

If that's justice here, it's what I fear,
It's barking up wrong tree.
If we don't end this awful trend,
We'll lose it all that's free.

And it frightens me that when I see
A stigma that's profound,
That gains support and much rapport
For people who's unsound!

If courtroom crews filled church's pews
Our problems would decrease.
Like flowing tides our precious prides
Then leads us back to peace.

So lets all pitch in with goal within
And toss the culprits out,
And vote those in whom we depend,
To bring this peace about!

❖❖❖❖❖❖❖❖

DAILY GRIND

Through the years and through the tears
I've seen the ups and downs.
I've fought the force and stayed the course
And tried to stay in bounds.

But it has been a hectic trend
In every daily way,
To meet the call, to fight appall
That comes with every day.

I rise up in the early morn
With planning on my mind,
On how to deal with worldly scorn
And with the daily grind.

It seems to me what's come to be,
Are people in a rut.
No one agrees, there's no appease,
With different views they strut.

The only answer I can see
Is turning to the Lord,
His love and care, His words to bear:
"Cease living by the sword!"

"THE STORM"

We, on the east coast don't particularly need a poem or verse reminding us of the problems and devastation caused by a hurricane, but this verse titled "The Storm" may at least contribute to our education of them and remind us how important it is to be aware of the damage they can bring and be prepared to deal with them safely.

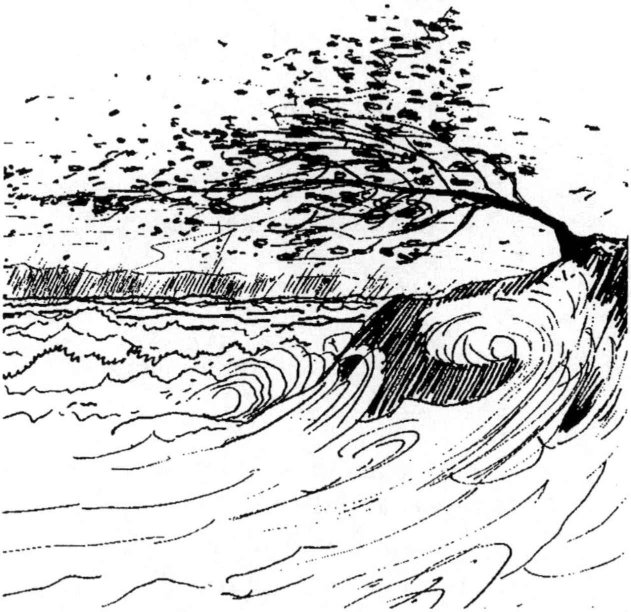

THE STORM

I am born and stand upon the sea
As a terrible and violent force
Of whirlwinds of a mass degree
Just spiraling on a course.

I have no special goal in mind,
I go where warm air leads,
To gain my strength I have to find
Warm water that heats my needs.

I'm called the most horrific storm
The world has ever known.
No greater force was ever born,
No greater winds have blown!

I am a killer from the sea.
I stay upon a verge.
I drown my site immediately
With my mighty water surge!

I am a mighty hurricane!
I romp the world at will,
Unleashing torrid winds and rain,
Upon the earth I spill!

I conquer all that's in my path,
I devastate and Kill!
I blast away with all my wrath
Before my winds come still.

I am the force that knows no bound,
Nor care what's in my wake.
I terrify all the life around
With all the furor I make.

I wash away, and tear away
What man has strove to build.
I'll blow it into disarray
Within a moments yield.

I'll flood his land, remove his sand,
And put him out to flee.
Run him out like no one can,
Except...the likes of me!

Although my winds are sometimes gone
I still retain a name;
I will form another spawn,
And I will storm again!

Here in the midst, some names I'll list,
But only just a few;
Was Danny, and Barry, Arthur
And Chris,
Cesar, Bob, and Andrew.

In '89 I had more fun
Where I dealt the mightiest
blow,
Upon the city of Charleston,
And my name was then Hugo.

I was Andrew named in '92,
In '93, I'm Stan.
In '96 I blasted through,
And my tag was labeled Fran.

My other names of hurricanes
Are Bertha and Isabel.
Wendy, Debby, and Helene
And the worst of all, Camille!

I left my marks upon the earth
With many more in store.
It's up to you folks, and all you're worth,
Take heed forevermore!

❖❖❖❖❖❖❖❖

When in our lives things don't seem to go right, and we have a tendency to rush or get too excited about the outcome of any particular situation, we need to slow down, better yet, stop and view the situation, and then proceed with our endeavor.

My following verses, "Slo Down", "Right Course," "Inner Voice" and "No Where To Go, But Up" are the best examples of advise I can suggest on what to do under stress.

SLO DOWN

There is a trait to nurture
Which behooves us to attain;
Patience is the virtue,
It will keep our problems plain!

For if we keep on rushing
Over life's long rocky lane,
It will all end up to nothing
Without solutions gain.

To slow down in our cadence
With long and deeper breaths,
Will give our lives more patience
To meet life's grueling tests!

For when our trumpets blow
And to glory we will shout;
We will have done it better, slow,
And it never wore us out!

❖❖❖❖❖❖❖❖

RIGHT COURSE

You do not need a college course
Or any school degree,
In learning how to show remorse
For all the bad we see.

It always seems that many folks
Deny when they are wrong.
They seem afraid their pride will fade
If they should "go along".

It's not uncouth to tell the truth
To avoid the verbal "web,"
Then what we weave won't be aloof,
But be dclight instead!

So don't hold back just let it go,
And let yourself be you,
And everyone will always know
Your heart is ever true!

❖❖❖❖❖❖❖❖

INNER VOICE

There's a deeper voice inside
That lends itself to guide;
But often leaves us all confused,
For in our oft' endeavors
When we doubt our shoulds and whethers,
Somebody usually gets abused!

So it's up to each deciding
That the problem may be chiding
When it shows it has this sort of ring;
So deny that inner voice
When in doubt about a choice,
Just give a smile and don't do anything!

For that little voice in there
Can sometimes be a dare,
Stemming from your mind's inner eye;
So in understanding this,
You will never be amiss,
And never need this voice to rely.

NO WHERE TO GO, BUT UP!

I'm the lowest on the "totem pole",
A long way from the top.
It's hard to see a distant goal
With a bottom view I got!

I've tried for years to make it up,
But much to no avail,
For long I thought "to fill my cup"
Meant "Fill it from a pail!"

I've been below a long, long while,
I'm used to all that weight
Which covered me beneath the pile,
That sealed my very fate.

But, someone has to bear the load
To hold the others up,
So glories there will get bestowed,
To "fill my brothers' cup".

But in the end I guess I'll win
For I'm their solid base,
For it is me whom they depend
To hold them up in place.

So when they hand diplomas out
And name the honor roll,
My name will be the first they shout
For low man on the pole!

"ALL THROUGH THE NIGHT"

I try not to think of my problem as growing older, although I suppose it's part of the process and I don't want to give the impression that I have insomnia and have a great deal of trouble sleeping. I guess I get enough sleep, it just seems to take a long time in getting it. I have a lot of enthusiasm about doing odd jobs around the house, and indulging in some sort of building project and take these ideas to bed.

Sometimes I'll sleep, then wake up thinking its morning, time to rise, only to discover it's 12:30 A.M. and I only slept a couple of hours. There seems to be many nights like that. The following verse describes an example of one of those nights.

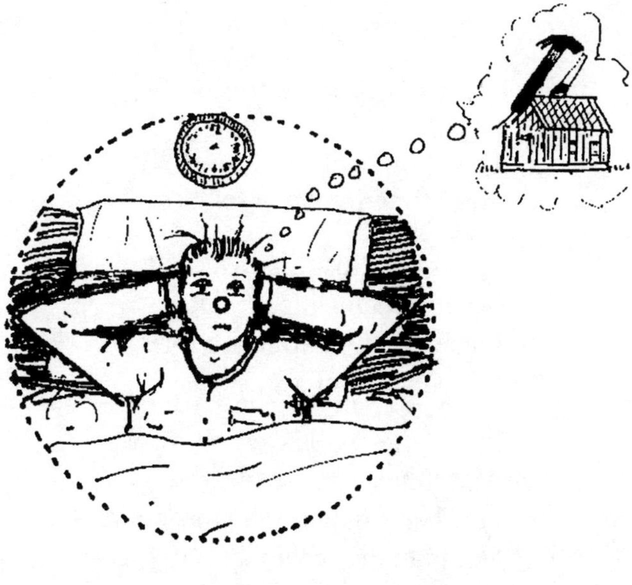

ALL THROUGH THE NIGHT

I'm already thinking of morning light
Before I go to bed;
Another night of toss and fight,
The length of it I dread!

For it often seems an endless fact
When crawling into the sack,
That I start my old pretending act
In trying to relax.

For I go to bed still planning themes
Of many chores I sight,
My thoughts continue scanning scenes
All through the entire night!

It's lying in bed that's killing me,
I just can't wait 'til dawn.
But by my clock it's only three,
Four hours more to yawn!

And life is getting shorter now,
The nights seem longer too,
To get more sleep, I must allow
More time for sleep to "brew".

I guess I'm just the restless type,
My life seems incomplete.
I need the time to make it right,
But can't if I'm asleep;

But in the end I'll get my rest
And things will be alright,
For then I plan to do what's best---
Not plan the whole darn night!

❖❖❖❖❖❖❖❖

"DAILY RUN"

I was employed over thirty three years by the C&O Railway system located in Newport News, Va. at the eastern end of the Peninsula. Since I lived in a westerly portion, I had to travel a distance of approximately 20 miles each shift I worked.

Now the railroad had different working hours, different crews, different duties, etc. and because of this nature, I sometimes would have to return to work after eight hours rest, but to make a long story short, it dawned on me one time that my entire life was spent traveling Jefferson Avenue and Warwick Boulevard.

So in my very short verse, "Daily Run", tells a lot about that time.

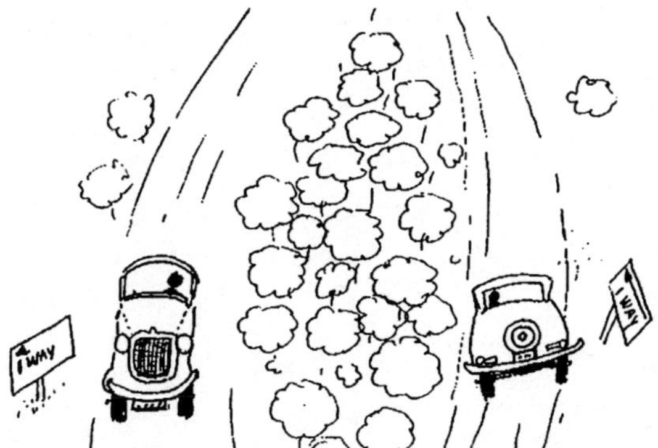

DAILY RUN

I've tread upon old Newport News
For nigh on fifty years.
I paid my dues, I've sang the blues,
I've seen the smiles and tears.

From home to work I carved a path
On each, a daily run;
On two vast avenues of wrath
Called Warwick and Jefferson.

I went up one and came back two
On every working day;
For 30 years I made it through
To C&O Railway.

To reach this yard and old shipyards,
That Newport News relied,
There came two added boulevards
Called Mercury and J. Clyde.

Now at this time comes thoughts in mind
Of how this place met change,
Of all the grind that I now find,
"Four lanes of tortures pain!!"

There appears to be another kind of turmoil existing in some peoples lives, and it's not new. I've seen it occur over the years as an outlet for some individuals to display their frustrations, their emotions and over what? Sports, yes, sports such as basketball, baseball, and football.

The soccer fans in Europe are famous for their outburst of excitement, anger and even death in their behavior. There is a trend in this country also for people to become too involved with their teams of choice winning or losing in the games they play, particularly in pro football.

IT'S ONLY A GAME

There is a trend in life within,
It's anger people show;
In game of life or game in strife,
By letting their tempers go!

I've heard it said that people dread
The very thought to lose;
That life itself goes on the shelf
When their team gets abused.

That it's their dream, a football team
Controlling their demands;
From morn to night they scratch and fight
With adversary fans.

They push and shove, shout high above,
And stomp upon the deck;
But when they lose they're in recluse,
And come a total wreck.

And in their dens when game begins
They want all others out;
So they can cuss or they can fuss
Or they can pout or shout!

And in the streets they air defeats
With fist fights all around,
And in the air, are gun shot blares
Supporting teams they're bound.

I heard of one who shot his son
Because of different view.
Now that's a shame to let a game
Come in between these two.

So on it goes with strife and woes,
Too many ills to name.
A football game or life the same,
It's ourselves we have to blame!

DOWN BUT NOT OUT

When you're way down in the "dumps"
and burdened with despair;
can you define the "lumps and bumps"
of things that got you there?

Are you for sure in certainty
just where to place the blame?
Will you decree for clarity
it's you, you have to name?

'Twas either you or something else
that makes your face so long,
so clean the shelf within yourself
will clear up what went wrong!

One needs to put his life on trial,
his own self be his judge,
and see his style without beguile,
to do away the grudge.

For if indeed someone cast "stones"
and broke your heart instead...
"it's sticks and stones that break the bones"
and words should never tread.

THE BOMB THAT BLEW ZEB AWAY

There is a tremendous population explosion in the world. That's a fact everyone should know by now. It seems that nothing is going to be done about it, unless like fictional "Old Zeb" we just find ourselves a lonely spot somewhere, although I'm sure it wouldn't be long before that space is crowded also. There are a lot of "Zebs" in this world who feel the walls are closing in on them, and with no disrespect intended, I use the character "Old Zeb" to illustrate this point.

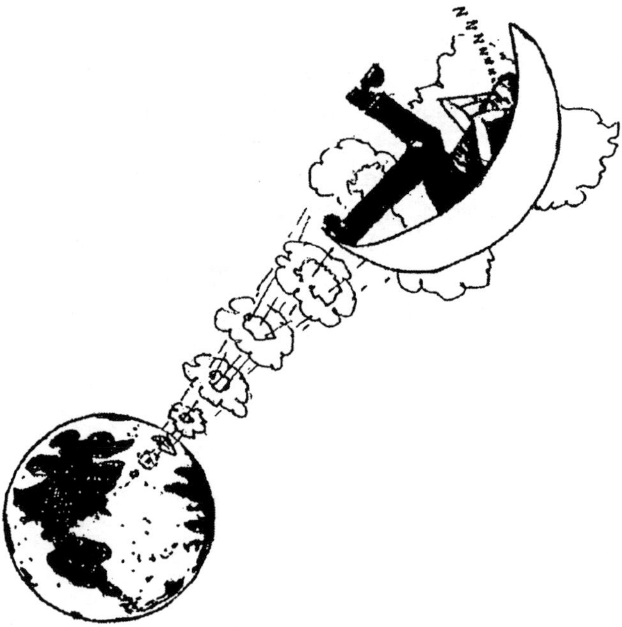

THE BOMB THAT BLEW ZEB AWAY

Out away from the busy town lies a fifty acre plot,
where "country" Zeb can be found nesting on his lot.
Now "country" Zeb, a good old soul, is liked by everyone.
He never went to school I'm told, but left a handsome sum.
I saw him on that sunny day shading beneath his tree;
stroking his beard of silver gray, smiling and feeling free.

I asked old Zeb if he'd explain just why he moved out here;
he said, "Cause of all the growin' pain, and all my cluster fear."
Then a twinkled eye, another sigh, and he wrinkled up his brow,
and commenced to say exactly why he came out here and how.
Now Zeb's grammar is left desired without an education;
so he wrote a poem to be inspired to give his explanation:

"I'm sic an' tarred of life in town, too many folks in ther'.
Too many autos all aroun' I caint hardly breethe the aere."
"We're the cast of some kinda blast, the fall out is us all!
We're multiplying'--too darn fast with no slo down a 'tall."
"A mass exploshun brings us here to liv on this grate land;
but we're congregatin too dawg near an' nobody can exspand."

"Thar aint no rore I hear no where, I don't see flames from it;
no smell of smoke or fumes in aere; but it just keeps gitten lit!"
"We're al'so strewn an' scattered 'bout just filling up a space,
but 'lotta space is runnin' out in one hel-uh-va pace!"
"Tha' populashun's explodin' on with sich a mitey force,
and there aint gonn be no zone if we don't stop in our corse."
"We, tha peeple, explodin' here, we're gonn'a keep dispersin,
on an' on, an' on I fear if we don't quit our rehersin!"
"Woodin it be nice to sackerfice an' ever' one just layed still?
All wood joy in pairodice. I know darn well I will!"

❖❖❖❖❖

ONE EYE MONSTER

Oh how I miss the good old days
when life was simple then.
I sit despaired in many ways
of this present living trend.
The problem is, I know it's true,
is this thing called TV.
It makes me mad, it makes me blue,
it has a spell on me.

It hasn't always been that way,
"it used to be a charm!"
But now it seems like every day
it's causing much alarm!
Because of that I'm in a trap,
my hope is to believe;
a better change in their format
will make me less naive.

It displays each others ills and woes
for back yard laundry lines;
to air their woes, their "dirty clothes,"
their filth of many kinds.
It airs their views, we can't reply;
we either watch and keep;
but if they're bent to spin and lie,
mine's going to the heap!

It controls our lives in many ways,
I often wonder now;
without TV those early days
of what we did, and how!
The Bible says that God has said:
"No other gods before me."
And that includes that awful dread,
a god they call TV!

❖❖❖❖❖

THE MOOSE HEAD POKER CLAN

'Twas five o'clock I came to knock at the rear of the moose head club.
Three raps on the door and then one more, and then some dude called "Bub",
peers outside through a hole inside to check my ticket stub.
When he sees it's me, he turns a key, and the door comes open wide.
I went inside the smoke-filled dive, and headed for the back room game,
through smoke and dust to fill my lust, where no one knows no shame.

Down the hall past the bathroom stall, to the last door on the right;
where I rapped once more like I did before, and they opened upon my sight.
We meet each day in the same old way and play on through the night;
with a game of wits 'til someone quits, a winner or loser's plight.
Poker is the game, and stud is the name, in a vicious way its played;
with "cut-throat" bets without any frets, and without any mercy gave.

I never do see any sympathy that comes from any man.
Our blood is cold and we have no soul when we play in this here clan!
I don't know why any normal guy is compelled to fill a void.
To work all day then lose his pay to ease his mind annoyed.
So I guess by now you know my brow has gathered a lot of sweat;
in dealing cards without regards for my families' strong regret.
But in this game I meet my fame, my ego's miles up high;
but when I lose...I'm in recluse and feel my end is nigh;
and through the years were many tears, just fighting a losing fight;
but back I went in anxious bent to win and end my plight.

For you always think you're on the brink of winning something great;
with aces down your heart will pound- for this pot to seal your fate;
but it often seems that some guy beams when his last card leaves the deck.
For it comes to mate his flush or straight, and makes me a total wreck!
When there is no gain I feel the pain and strive with new desire;
to win so bad what I once had, then douse my gambling fire!
But all us men are hard within and won't give up our ploy;
each man is steel with a stubborn will, to reach some height of glory.

Through all the maze and smoking haze, our piercing eyes go daunting,
to find a way to make all pay, by bluffing and in flaunting,
but we gather here together whether luck is good or not;
all our fever won't last forever, because time will cure this lot!
I always hope not to be a dope, and some "flash in the pan"
but its not old news, that I always lose when I play in the moose head
clan!

❖❖❖❖❖

A WORD TO THE WISE

All my life I've been a procrastinator. I'm not proud of that -- in fact, I don't think I knew its real meaning until recent years. I've always involved myself in all sorts of activities as I came along. On everything I set out to do I would try and give it 100 percent. I never really concentrated in any one particular thing. Sports, art, carpentry and music were just a few things that I did well. However, in my later years, I began to regret that I did not expand. In the following poem, "A Word To The Wise." I explain a little further.

A WORD TO THE WISE

A genuine plan follows every man until his time o'er,
And with each one the chances come to knock upon his door.
I heard mine knocked, but left it locked on many a splendid goal.
So here I am like a hornless ram, with my future still on hold!
So I'm in a net and have regret, my life is nigh on spent;
And I'll recall some falls I met and where the efforts went.
If it was great to procrastinate, to cite this trend I guess,
First place ribbons by the largest crate would at my door step rest!

For in the past I saved for last many goals I dreamed,
And always went no where fast in same old ways it seemed.
I loved to hear an auctioneer and like him wished to be;
Hear him with a voice unclear, "one dollar, two dollar, three!"
But I must say along the way this task did not occur,
And to this day I feel dismay due to that defer.
I visioned me on open sea as rugged captain bold,
But wasn't meant for me to be in this dramatic role.

So I set sails on other trails, one a college grad,
But in my sight there was no might and this dream wasn't had.
Procrastinate! What a debate! It's the worst ill known to man,
But it's the thing I do best and shows an also ran!
I wound it up a railroad man where thirty years I spent;
Almost half a life time span just wondering where it went!
And around my home (I still don't own) I'm loaded with many a chore;
I work my fingers to the bone getting no where as before.

So don't be like me, set your will free and give it all you got.
Pursue your goals at high degree, should be your lasting plot;
And don't delay your dreams today for tomorrow may never come.
Reach your height with vigor ways to better jobs well done.
And after all is said and done and your life is fixed by fate;
Did your successes add up - none, Because you chose to wait?

❖❖❖❖❖

Since retirement, I have developed a very strong urge to express certain views and opinions about moralistic values in the form of poetry and verse. I always believed in the values represented in them. As a father, I tried to instill these qualities in my children; although, I learned by my own life's earlier experiences that nobody is perfect and the standards I present in most of my poems are not always easy. The following poems merely convey what I believe to be the very best standards that people should strive to live by.

EYES OF TRUTH

Some folks plan to scheme and scam with intent to deceive,
but unaware, the deeds they dare, others just don't believe!
Except for those who undergoes the practice to pretend,
but "every row of seed they sow" will never grow a stem.
Where sly folks go they often show themselves as who they're not,
but in due time they'll surely find that no one "bought their plot!"
They're known for their iniquity; with egos in account.
Where their wrong trait leads on to hate, and too much woe will mount.
Here are examples that explain about this sort of thing,
about a man in his golf game and what his actions bring.
He struck the ball from off a tee, but errant was his aim,
his golf ball hits a big oak tree, and the golf course got the blame!

Now, his ball was found way "out of bound," but pretense came to be,
... and since he saw no one around, he thought none else would see.
His second shot, came to a stop against a fence too high,
with obvious gall he lifts the ball to improve on his bad lie.
So he plays on, the way he's prone, to reach the final green,
he holes the cup with his fourth putt, and still thinks no ones seen;
for on his card he marks it parred, a <u>4</u> that none will see.
A score of course that brings reward, but <u>10</u> it ought to be!
Now he may play alone in golf and also in his life,
but the saying goes "to each his own," will bring this guy much strife.
Here's a thought that I've been taught; it goes along like this:
"Man must learn to love himself to gain eternal bliss,
but love dear God before all else, for that's what God insists!"
And here's a fact and not a pun: I think may need review,
that you're not fooling anyone when you're only fooling you,
that just as true as rising sun, to yourself you must be true,
and if you follow this along, and do the best you can,
Then you'll never be seen as wrong, in view of any man.

BATTLE CRY

It's not a war that's fought on sea nor one where caissons roll;
not one with gun or cannon's roar nor shells that rockets dole;
but in the minds and hearts of men, the battleground - their soul!
There's been wars and rumors of wars, this one, the greatest fought!
a battle within the bosom of man and web in which he's caught!
He struggles each day to find a way to gain his freedom sought.

A war of sin with women and men, the war zone is their soul.
The games they play with reckless joy are played without a goal.
It's been on-going since winds been blowing, a story often told.
This old trend glides like ocean's tides that laps upon its shore;
and on man speeds with thoughtless deeds 'til he can go no more,
but it will last 'til lives have passed, that strayed therein before.

How many times can people sin without a thought of care?
How many times to ask the Lord to save them from their fear?
A road too rough that they made tough, they need to be sincere.
To find the will to bow and kneel without the fear of shame,
and ask dear God to come and fill their hearts in Jesus' name.
To stop deceiving and start believing that Christ died not in vain!

Still all the while others will file along a sinners trail,
they too, will lose with sex and booze and put their life for sale!
They will go on 'til they atone within their private hell!
And so beneath each silent voice are yearning battle cries,
and in each burning breast some inner spirit dies;
so therein lies the battle ground where all their hope relies.

Now who am I to say what's best or anyone to rate?
"Because I left that lonely path before it was too late;
and now I feel, that I've been healed by God's true lasting faith!"

❖❖❖❖❖

TROUBLED HEART

Sometime, somewhere, a body must start,
If they're in some deep trouble within,
To remove the turmoil of a burdened heart
By asking God to forgive them for sin.
Some look to the world and it's treasures sought
In hopes of fulfilling their gain,
But they will live on without any thought
Of the cause of their strife and pain.
Their search is on going for riches and fame
And yes, some have reached their goals;
But are they aware from whence they came
And the forces that played in their roles?
Is it God that is absent from their heart and mind
As they go through their life of grind?
And is it the devils drive in which they find
Themselves in their terrible bind?

But the strain of life is upon us all
And is not limited to just the rich,
For many a wealthy one stands tall
By using God's post to hitch.
'Cause God doesn't care how much money we earn
As long as it's honest and clean,
By instilling in us His foundation firm
Is living His precious theme!
So friends, if you're bothered in any way
And you're famous and wealthy or poor,
Take all the problems you have each day
And unload 'em at heavens door;
And the Lord is there to receive them with care,
Which He will dispose at will;
When in heaven we come to greet Him there,
We will have paid Him in full, our bill!

❖❖❖❖❖

RIGHT TURN

A crossroad comes in every life
Where people choose between;
The proper route that ends their strife,
Or way they've always seen.
And many will reach that crossing road
With dead end straight ahead,
Carrying a heavy burden load,
And ill will that was bred.

For many a man has gone astray
With many a wicked deed,
Stepped on toes along the way,
And not a heart would bleed;
Some griped a lot in traffic's snare,
And when the lights were red.
Smiled not upon a friendly stare,
But cast out frowns instead!

Or spatting with their friends and foe
And especially family,
They wonder now which way to go
To reach tranquillity.
So I suggest at the intersect
You have one choice of two,
Upon your past if you'll reflect,
Turn right, for life anew.

❖❖❖❖❖

A HUMAN COMEDY

I have no way of knowing how many other folks see and feel like I do about the nature of our life in this country. I have a tendency to notice how things play out in everyday occurrences, especially on television and the news in general.

Right now, I think there is just too much controversy about everything and too much polarization in the minds and views that are displayed on a daily basis. It can be a little disturbing, I think, if one has a tendency to take sides. I guess I'm speaking generally about politics, although I see a lot of other activities that bother me as well - like court trials where there is a great sense of injustice prevailing. Also, it's shown in matters of racial differences. I've come to look at the situation as a huge play being played out before the country where the actors themselves don't even realize they're in it.

This, I believe, adds to the "joke" elements displayed in life. It's what I refer to as the "Human Comedy" followed by the "Right Tune" which suggests what everyone can do about life's controversies.

A HUMAN COMEDY

There is a "big show" going on. I've got a front row seat!
I view the action, hear its drone with every sounding beat:
from television in my home, from out upon the street.
I watch the actors in their play acting out their theme;
observing how and what they say, and what they really mean.
Sometimes I laugh, sometimes I cry, and times I pine or pout,
because of things that go awry or how the scenes play out.

The leading actors in this play are usually folks of fame;
we can see them every day on TV in their game,
like congress folks who polarize, no progress have they made.
They are the clowns shown in disguise, are images displayed.
Other actors in this show are folks like you and me;
standing on the side lines though,we're still in this melee.
The funny part about this play it doesn't seem to end.
The plot continues on each day with interesting trend.

Some folks agree, some disagree,some take a different view.
The biggest problems that I see, is seeing nothing new!
And yet, I know what you will say; "This is the land of free,
that it's the good old U.S.A., our right to disagree".
But what I see disturbing me sings not a pleasant song,
'cause folks are firm in their decree, but really know they're wrong.

So goes the show it must go on, just play the daily scenes,
the final act is yet to come with many plots and schemes.
the final act will be a fight where people come to band,
to fill their roles with all their might so all can understand.
Where cheers go up for those who're right, hurrahs for those who're
bound;
to solve the problems of our plight then ring the curtain down!

❖❖❖❖❖

THE RIGHT TUNE

I'm weary of all the spoils of life.
I'm tired of all the gloom.
Sick of all the talk of strife
And lectures of our doom!

I'm leery of the TV shows
That dwell on woes and crimes,
And all the violence it bestows
Upon our children's minds!

I'm disgusted with the media press
For distorting many facts,
Just plain angry with the carelessness
Of our politician's acts.

So what's the answer to my woe?
The choice comes down to this:
I can either stay the status quo
or wave a good-bye kiss!

A better choice I've come to see,
I believe without a doubt,
Is tune in only what's good for me
And tune the evil out!

HOW TO QUIT SMOKING LESSON

I started smoking cigarettes when I was about 10 years old. As a kid I would hide away so nobody could see me. At that age I felt guilty about what I was doing, also back in those days there wasn't the notion that cigarettes were harmful to one's health. Of course, today we know this is true, and since I quit smoking I have developed an actual feeling of nausea when I'm around cigarette smoke.

When I came out of the Air Force in 1952, I smoked an average of three packs a day - and as one might imagine, I wasn't feeling too well back then. I had lost a lot of weight and became determined to do something about it. I developed a plan that would help me quit, and I put it into operation.

It actually worked. Although it wasn't easy, I did manage to quit. It was 35 years from that time to 1987 when I underwent open-heart surgery, yet doctors attributed the problem to my smoking habit. The poem, "How to Quit Smoking Lesson," which may sound more like a "sermon," is the actual plan I used in my endeavor.

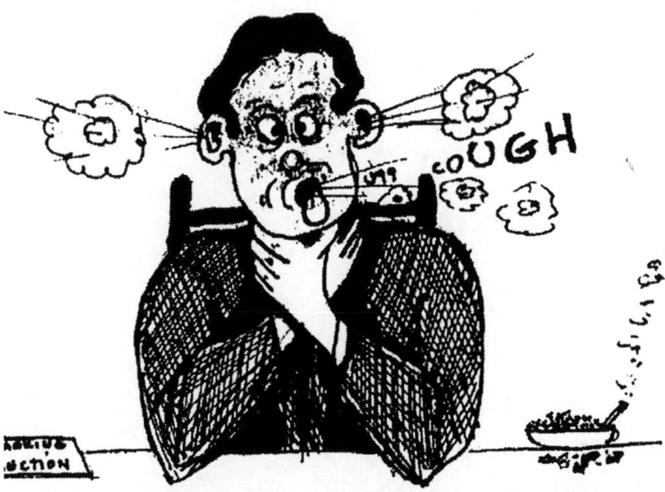

HOW TO QUIT SMOKING LESSON

So you want to quit smoking do you? Well, pull up a chair and sit down there
and I'll tell you what to do, with rules you have to bear.
You'll come to see what's best to be, and you will quit for sure.
It worked for me in '53, and brought about my cure!
No rougher puffer ever born, I smoked three packs a day.
No tougher war in me was torn while puffing them away!
From dawn to night with every pack I drawed 'em 'til I spat;
From night to dawn with cough and hack my taste buds all ways flat!
So just relax and keep your packs, and while I tell it through,
You will know the facts of things that you must dare to do!
Now listen up don't interrupt this main and vital part:
Just one big puff should be enough to get you on the start,
You train your brain to see a strain in that one breath of smoke...
With vision that its not in vain for you to have a stroke!
Next, don't hesitate to set a date for smoking to decease...
But smoke those things until it brings the date when you release.
Now in this trying time of dread keep smoking to down size--
Smoke 'em 'fore you go to bed and smoke 'em when you rise.
But now you say: "I want to quit" well, I'll get on to that!
But in your fit you must admit that you're a smoking sap!
Now keep on puffing every day with malice in your smoke,
With every breath---you just think - death. This should cure your croak.
Now don't forget, your cigarette is only just a crutch.
It adds more fret to your regret - while piling up the butts.
Now, check how far on calendar your trial time has so reached -,
And let's just say you're 'bout midway before your time will cease --
So on you go with puff and blow but cuss 'em with each breath -
Cuss 'em with all vile you know then give 'em kiss of death!
Now comes the date you face your fate your nerves are on the brink;
Either open, mate, or close the gate. Either swim now or you sink!

But now don't sweat and please don't fret - because a "shrink" once said:
"When body and your mind has met; 'tis better alive than dead!"
I'm betting on you, you'll pull it through, like me, you got much pride...
If I can do it, so can you...so don't go run and hide!
With retrospect you now inject a will into your mind;
You can't reject the side effect, a strength that you will find.
Its last trial night and do not light..... but, crush that cigarette!
And tomorrow's might will end your plight, 'cause you just can't help but quit!

❖❖❖❖❖

CALL OF THE WILD

In today's society we are living in a very disturbing time. It seems as though everything is going "haywire" and completely out of control. The crime rate is running rampant and the permissiveness allowed in our schools and court systems is alarming! I say this because I've often felt anger and despair in what I see going on in our country today.

While I don't intend to shoot myself over it, I'll continue to express what I think is the right way to live. The following three poems, "Call Of The Wild," "Living Gone Awry," and "Holiday Season," make the point of our problems today.

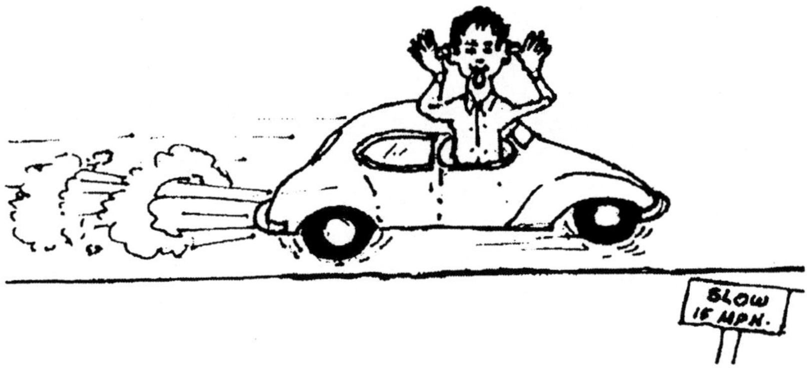

CALL OF THE WILD

This is a story of "Call Of the Wild," and not the epic I read as a child.
It is not a novel about Eskimo dogs, but cars and crooks called Highway Hogs!
A war in a jungle right here on our street. We must fear for our lives each day we meet.
Hogs use their vehicles like missiles of war and fire them at us on roads of tar.
We are forced to defend with all of our skill, or become victims of their urge to kill!
We try to steer clear from these clods so riled, the rogues that enter the "call of the wild"!

A drunken driver in search of his lust did fly away in a cloud of dust, and without caring, without any heed, ran through a red light with tremendous speed.
He left us in shock with thunder-like roar, his foot on the pedal, flat on the floor.
This pickled brain idiot in his lifestyle is playing his role in "call of the wild"!

A saddened fellow betrayed by his girl decided to let his feelings unfurl, so on his seat he placed his butt, now behind this wheel we see a loose nut.
Away he sped into thick of traffic like a rodeo cowboy after his maverick!
No glimmer of hope or even a smile, this guy just joined the "call of the wild"!

These jerks believe they are kings of the roads and view all others as swampland toads,
that nobody can be on the highway but them, as they wear out their tires from rim to rim.
So here are the people with ego much, for they are compelled to strut their stuff.
Their use of their cars that is a crutch to show everybody that they are tough.
Filled with conceit, and many are vile eager to respond to the "call of the wild"!

The problem we have is we cannot exist among the road hogs out there in our midst,
We can only do the best that we can 'til enough cops can enforce a ban.
You may recall this sort of event, like this one coming to mind,
that when on a trip where much time was spent, some fool approaches behind.

He comes as fast as lightning's blast... and displays a one-finger sign!
For miles I saw a clear lane ahead, and yet he forces me over,
not passing way out, instead, he cut in from of my Nova.
This clown...traveled his way up the road where an eighteen-wheeler waxed this toad.
He joined the stats where many are filed; of those hogs who chose the "call of the wild!"

Not all who drives meets this description, for we join hands to fill this prescription,
and that is to drive with safety and pride to our destinations where we arrive alive.
Share the road with courtesy smile, avoiding trouble in "call of the wild"!

Some other factor that enters equation, and that is the crime wave crippling our nation.
They are kin in ways, and neither are mild, the crooks and the hogs in "call of the wild."
When they aim their shot, could be one of two: either their auto or "thirty-two!"
It isn't safe especially at night, they just shoot for fun and then take flight!

Call it a drive-by, a cowardly deed. They just get their kicks, an ego to feed.
Don't know their reason, this concrete rebel, he will meet his Maker, not God, but the devil!
What ever we own, thieves can't stand it. They gun their way in and demand it.

They impede our lives with arrogance and gall. We show our distrust with anxious appall.
We fear for our lives, our children as well, for even our schools are going through hell!
I really try hard to understand what's happening in our land,
'cause found behind the bars are we, while murderers go roaming free!

No greater battle than on our street, no better lesson than "run and retreat."
No greater jungle between Congo ad Nile that equals this scare in "call of the wild"!
There must be some power more powerful than us that can put a halt to this terrible fuss.
A Great Hand must come from Heaven above to stop all this hate and replace it with love,
Return us to glee, humor, and smile, and vanquish forever this "call of the wild"!

LIVING GONE AWRY

What else can go awry in this everyday rat race?
What on earth can change our hustle, bustle pace?
For every time we turn around we run into a bind.
We contact many people with some of them unkind.
You meet them in a market square when in some line you stand;
Someone in the rear may blare a very harsh demand!
"Hurry up and write your check," they yell out with a lash.
"You're showing a lot of disrespect not paying your bill with cash."
"Can't you see that sign up there that reads no "checks express"
And pay with cash your grocery fare for items ten or less?"
Which one are you I ask standing in that line?
Are you the one they're shouting at, or one that shouts behind?

And when you're in a market store (choose anyone in town),
Bargain hunters by the score are surely to be found;
And many folks are rushing all around the place;
When announced that a sale is on they stampede in a race,
And if you're trampled in your flight escaping to the door;
Control your fright with all your might, just lay and hug the floor!
There're many times when people shop to buy the right supply,
But sometimes ends up in a flop, and often goes awry!
For when they get their treasures home they find some faulty things,
And this brings on an anguish moan for trouble that it brings.
The problem is, you often find, they're cheap but cost a lot,
And you wind up in a waiting line, a short line it is not!

In one line a woman waited, one hour was her belief,
And when she reached the front--she stated: "I've lost my cash receipt!"
This brought on snarls and chaos from others in the line,
'Cause they're waiting for the store boss for an OK he must sign!
Finally the boss appears and some folks start to curse,
For he has them all expressing sneers by emptying out her purse!
Then at last he's satisfied he's thorough as could be,
That in this case she had not lied, he then returned her fee.

Now pale and wan with smileless face she said to this guy:
"This is such a hectic place, no more from you I'll buy!"
So on her way back out the store to find her route back home,
She tripped and fell and hit the floor and could have broke a bone!
"What else can go awry?" she hissed, as she withered there in pain.
"What have I done to deserve all this? I'm not the one to blame!"

And out upon the busy roads are vehicles all around;
And nobody cares, sees or knows exactly where they're bound!
It's a mad, mad rush to be the first upon the scene arriving,
And in one cloud of speed they burst in ways of reckless driving.
We are going fast to go no where in walking, run or drive,
And its bringing all so much despair, some won't arrive alive!
Because we're all too busy folks to slow ourselves with care;
We all end up with dizzy strokes and can't go anywhere!
We just don't take enough of time especially when we're high,
And you can bet your only dime that something goes awry!

❖❖❖❖❖

HOLIDAY SEASON

Today is Thanksgiving day and rush to Christmas starts.
Tomorrow the crowds will make their way to all the malls and marts.
It's labeled as the busiest time of all the entire year,
and multitudes will stand in line for bargains far and near.
The streets will jam with many cars with sounds of every horn,
and greatest spars of all street wars begins tomorrow morn.

From every home, they'll look and roam - to fill each parking space.
Through every hall and stall they'll comb, in pace that comes a race!
The malls fill up humanity, with thousands on the round,
looking at all gifts to see if discounts can be found!
This surge will last through Christmas Eve and on to Christmas Day,
does anyone, do you believe, stop long enough to pray?

It seems sometimes that Christmas joy has lost its truthful meaning,
where business shows commercial's ploy, which needs a thorough cleaning!
So recognize its Christ's birthday and gifts are just tradition,
that we should give our thanks and pray, which is our main condition.
So take out "X" and put Christ in, then "Christmas" truly shows--
continue in this grateful trend and joy in yuletide flows!

IDEALS

VIRGINIA IS FOREVER

We sing aloft our praises,
As pride within us raises
Of the land we love and call our
own;
From the mighty Shenandoah
To the sands of Eastern Shore,
Virginia is forever our dear home.

Where from her trees and bowers
We breathe the dogwood flowers,
Where the red birds make their presence known;
And lovers make their claim
Where history makes its name,
Virginia is forever that dear home.

Where folks of all the races
Can depend on her embraces,
And she brings much hope to those alone.
Where happiness is felt
Here in the Commonwealth,
Virginia will forever be our home.

When springtime fills her mountains,
And rain drops fill her fountains,
The apple blossoms then come fully grown;
And the nights are cool and crisp
'Til the morning sun is kissed,
In Virginia, which forever is our home.

So Virginia is forever
For everyones endeavor,
And we rise to praise and set the tone;
For opportunity
In a land where we are free,
In Virginia, our dear and blessed home.

❖❖❖❖❖❖❖❖

"MY FINEST HOUR"

I landed a job in 1955 with the C&O Railway Co. It came at a special time in my life when I could have easily gone another direction, so I feel much dedication for that.

I loved the nature of the particular work that made the railroad operate, which "got in my blood", so to speak. The verse "My Finest Hour" depicts my thoughts about that activity.

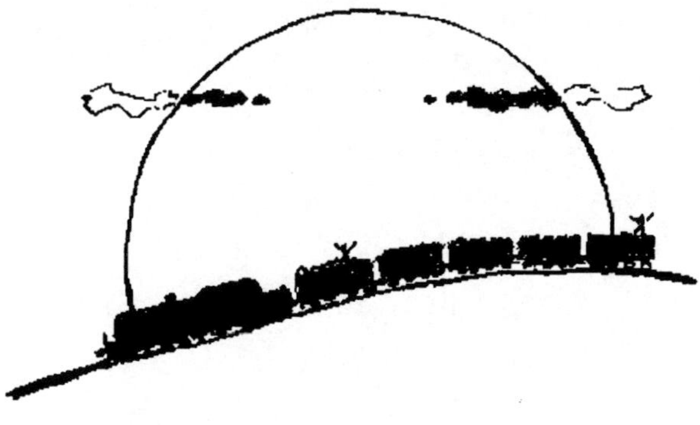

MY FINEST HOUR

There was no better job around
That matched the C&O.
It was a hallmark that I found
In years of long ago.

It came in just the "nick of time"
When I was down and out.
It made my life again sublime
And lit my darkened route.

But that was in the far gone by
And all those times are spent.
The memories that I hold so high
Would fill a circus tent.

But at those times I never knew
'Twas memories being made,
And many friendships that were true,
Are ones that never fade.

What I recall reminds us all
Of railroad sounds and sights;
To toil in heat, or cold, or squall,
In rain or snowy nights.

I'm not the only one I think
Who has a yarn to spin,
For many folks still in the pink
Was there with me back then.

To all my pards of old rail yards.
In downtown Newport News,
I give to you my best regards
For times we spent on crews.

We coupled cars, pulled lever bars,
And lined the switches straight;
We coupled hose on all the cars
When making up the freight.

We tied the brakes we opened gates
We worked the many piers;
We opened locks, turned angle cocks
And signaled engineers.

We rode atop, but walked a lot,
And pulled a many pin;
We spotted cranes, we made up trains,
And worked the old coal bin.

We flagged the roads to place the loads,
And pull the empties too;
We worked the yards, the car float barge
With many a midnight crew!

We had to know which way to go,
And where the cars to hold,
Or lift the skates, or loosen brakes
When off a hill to roll.

We had to use and not abuse
The hand held radio,
To signal crews to make our moves,
To make our system go!

And everytime we walked a track
To make a certain cut,
We always had to call for slack
To get the pin pulled up.

Now here I find myself serene
On twilights golden tower;
Looking backward on a dream
Which was "my finest hour."

❖❖❖❖❖❖❖❖

"WALK"

In the past several years, walking for fun and exercise has probably reached an all time high. Of course the weight and cholesterol factors have played a great part in its popularity. I know from experience because walking was prescribed for me by doctors. I found something more in walking, to me it was resting, yes resting, the kind the mind gets when you feel really good inside. I get that when I'm out walking. Sometimes I feel like breaking into a dead-run, but I suspect that's what would happen if I tried that! In any case, the following verse, "Walk", tells how I feel about walking.

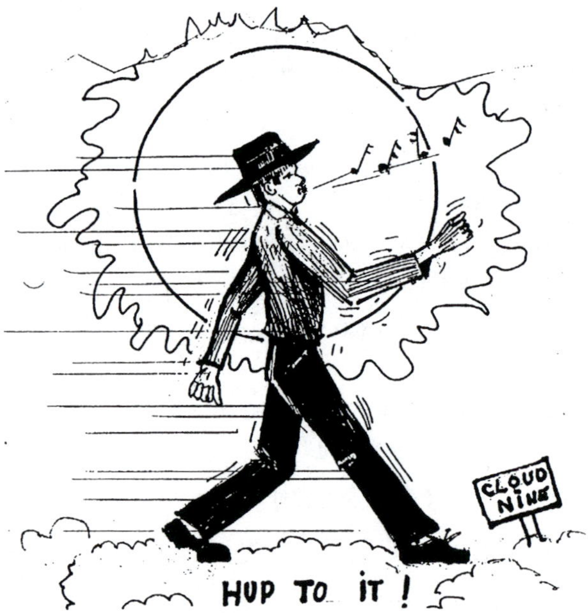

WALK

Go pick'em up and set'em down
And walk some every day;
Walk to work, walk to town,
And walk what ever may!

Walk, walk, walk, Oh how great it feels
To go outside and stride;
And walk away the daily meals
That we just stored inside.

And walk away your troubles too,
And hit the trails today;
And walk, and walk, and walk 'til you
Have walked your fears away!

And when you walk, walk down some street
You never walked before;
And watch for signs and things to meet
That walking has in store.

For sights you see come closer here
Not seen from any car.
A smile, a handshake from someone near,
'Tis better to me by far!

And see the things that comfort brings
When walking to and fro,
Pretty houses, folks in swings,
Maybe someone you know!

So go and walk, and walk, and walk,
And walk your life around,
And with you take this cadence talk;
"Pick'em up and set'em down".
("And hup to it, when you do it")

❖❖❖❖❖❖❖❖

"A LESSON IN HUMILITY"

I learned long ago that you can't get too "high on your horse" when it comes to every day activity or in most cases when you're competing in some sort of sporting events. We all like to feel we're on top of the world when we come to realize we do a particular thing better than most folks. I was taught my lesson early in life by a small country school basketball team named Dixon High School located near Jacksonville, NC in 1948.

I was a member of a varsity high school team in Wilmimgton, NC, who dominated the eastern conference league over a period of several years, and like everyone who supported us, we were in "high cotton" as the saying went.

Feeling cocky and overbearing is probably putting it mildly. Even the newspaper reporter that covered our games was so confident we would win this particular game, that he wrote a column of our having won, and even adlibed results of how we did it without showing up for the game. Which, of course added to our embarrassment the next morning. To put it mildly, "Dixon took us down a peg."

So it was that cold night in January 1948 that reminded me to write this following verse, "A Lesson in Humility".

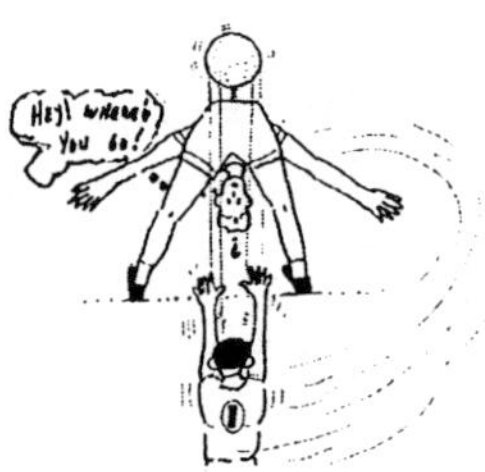

A LESSON IN HUMILITY

There is a fact that's pending of a tale that has no ending,
And it 's always when you think you can't be beat
In daily work or play, or in a contest fray,
A lesser one will come with your defeat.

This tale that I'm revealing, to me is so appealing,
Although this act of fate occurred to me;
That once in '48 these facts I now relate,
How I learned a lesson in humility!

In basketball we won, we were rated number one.
For two years we didn't lose a game.
As a member I would beam on this mighty high school team,
And never lose again was our main aim.

But for a special treat to make their day complete,
We went one night to play this country school;
We went there for their awe to prove that we weren't raw,
And to let them see that we were great and cool!

We were cool alright 'cause the temperature that night
Was as cold as a pawn broker's heart;
And when we entered in their small and icy gym,
The thermometer was reading down to naught!

Where there we had to hov' by an old "pot belly" stove
To warm and thaw our fingers to respond,
And the referees came in to bade the game begin
With overcoats and muffs that they had donned.

And when their team came out, there rose a hearty shout
From the sixty-seven people in the stands,
And their players looked so small in their uniforms and all,
And not once did they come and warm their hands.

And when the game began, with the basketball they ran,
And they looked like they never played adept,
But every time they shot, and it seemed an awful lot,
And every time it went right through the net!

For now I must admit that they gave our team a fit,
And never once again I'll take for granted;
That little country team who blew our self esteem,
Who gained our respect that they demanded.

And now I see it clear there is a message here,
That no matter how skilled you come to be;
That if you're great or small or even short or tall,
There's always someone better than you or me.

"RISE AND SHINE"

I suppose the older one gets, especially if they're retired, are always looking for something to fill their time, so in order to pump myself up in the morning I start this process of finding something to do that makes me feel good and active. In the following verse "Rise and Shine" are my suggestions on some of these.

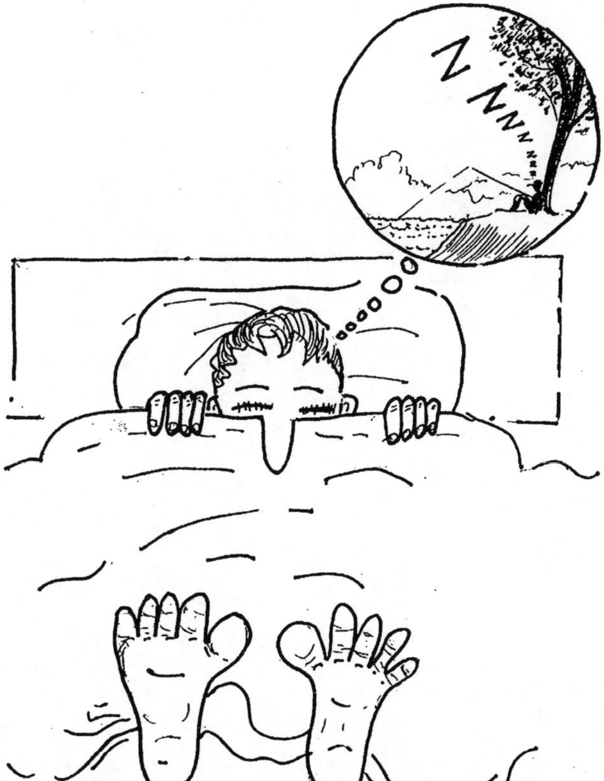

RISE AND SHINE

When you rise up in the morning,
Are there thoughts of what to do?
Like doing chores with bliss adorning
That makes your life feel new.

How 'bout jobs that bring rewards,
Those keeping your mind in peace,
Like mowing the grass and water the yards,
Or walking your dog on leash,

Or building a simple blue bird house,
Or painting your wood shed red.
Getting your spirits to really arouse
By painting your house instead!

A thousand things that joy here brings,
Just waiting for your cool hand,
So remove your weight on those inner
springs
And rise and do what's grand!

If you will perform what I suggest,
Then I know you're not a dub;
'Cause they're the deeds we love the best,
So welcome to our club!

OUR CLASS OF '52

We come to the door of memory hall
To raise the banners high.
We stand together one and all
To hail the sweet gone by.

We gather here in a joyous state
To praise the gold and blue;
To share the memories that relate
To our class of '52!

From high school days in Newport News
Where pride was our best guide,
With a brilliant show of golds and blues,
To anniversary 45!

Here, within these walls of memory hall
We raise our glasses high;
A toast to those whom we recall,
Our memory will never die;
Of the image of the ones we see
Will live forever fond.......
Miss Gildersleeve, T.O. Keesee,
Coaches, Powers and Julie Conn.
George McIntosh, our leader true,
Our coach called "Cowboy" Raine,
With these names and others too,
Will in our hearts remain.

Our memory soars as it goes indoors
To the busy halls we knew,
Chattering, smiling in gleeful noise
Of students passing through.

We're treading the way to each classroom
Just thrilled with life's good pleasures,
Thinking not of any future doom,
Only of it's precious treasures!

Now here we stand in a future realm
Emerging from a distant time,
Perseverance was the guiding helm
That made our friendships bind.

We pray for the loved ones passed away,
As classmates we did bond;
They too, in our hearts will always stay
As we strive to carry on.

So with heartfelt care of the thoughts we hold,
A toast to all who's here.
"Cheers to us, to the BLUE and GOLD,
'Til we meet in a future year!"

This poem was written on behalf of my wife Bobbie and her fellow classmates of Newport News High Schools Class of 1952 in honor of their 45th reunion.

❖❖❖❖❖❖❖❖

"A CLOUDY EXAMPLE"

I was very young, about six years old I think, when my Mom described the summer billowing clouds one day, telling me to view those patterns and formations, and I would see figures, faces of people, Santa Claus, etc.

Since then I've done it many times, even today. I don't think there's a person living that hasn't done it at one time or another. In any event, the short verse "Cloudy Example" explains this simple procedure.

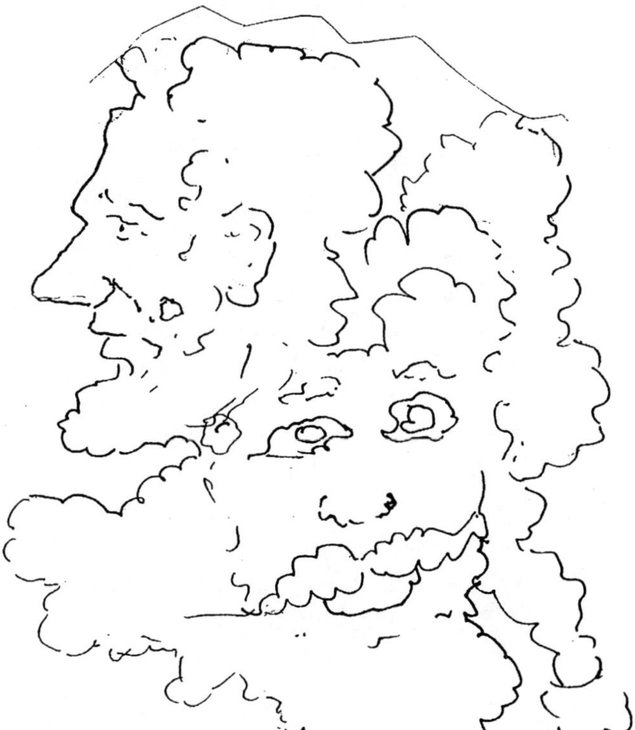

A CLOUDY EXAMPLE

Have you ever stood in the great outdoor
And peered at a cloudy sky?
And looked for a face you've known before
In a cloud that formed on high?

Well, I did as a kid as we played this game,
And we had to name who's who,
So the winner came when he came to name
The names of the most he knew.

It's a lot of fun 'cause I always won
On a fact of the strangest thing;
That no matter where in a cloud that sprung,
Is a face my mind would bring.

Now don't deny, simply go and try
On a fleecy cloudy day,
And start by thinking of Abraham Lincoln,
Then scan the clouds array.

I'll swear to you, from outta' the blue
You'll know that his face appeared;
By his big bow tie and tall hat too,
And the length of his hairy beard.

I've given an ample, foregone sample,
The next step's up to you--,
To test my sample for your example
To find my finding true;
That from here on out you'll have no doubt
Of the tale I've told to you!

"THE OLD GRIST MILL"

The grist mills are of course relics today. Those that are left have probably been restored and preserved. What a beautiful reminder of the life that surrounded that activity! They are indeed antiques of life. They represent a kind of serenity that can effect all who see them.

In my poem "The Old Grist Mill" describes a version of that activity. The next following short poem, "My Own Grist Mill" is merely a reverent feeling inspired by the first poem.

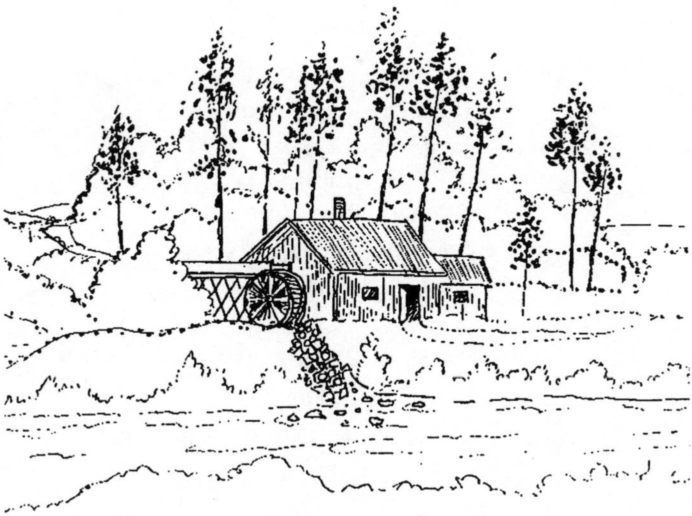

THE OLD GRIST MILL

Ah, there it sits upon that hill
Beneath a row of pines;
The last remains of Grandpa's mill,
A relic of early times.

See, below those boulders there
Where once the water flowed?
The old turn wheel of yesteryear
Is weathered, decayed, and bowed.

As I view this quaint old spot
A cloak of calm prevails;
Reminds me of the joys I got
And all the pleasant tales.

My memory eye goes there inside
Back when the grind wheel turned;
Where corn meal from its hull was pried
When on the grind stone churned.

And I recall from long ago
When I was only ten;
Gramps, hitching up his cart to tow
With a mule hooked, and then;

There across the doorway sill
In and out he'd dart;
Carrying sacks of ground corn meal
To stack up on the cart.

Then, after loading the cart up full
He'd climb up there on top;
And yank the reigns on that old mule
To go to his next stop;

Perhaps to some old market place
Or to a baker's shop,
But I recall most every case
'Twas bread for my Grandpop!

Well, there he goes beyond the hill,
He's gone and out of view;
All pleasant thoughts that linger still
Of the times that I once knew.

So there upon that lofty hill
My lovely landmark rests;
A lasting memory of this mill
Back when it was its best!

❖❖❖❖❖❖❖❖

MY OWN GRIST MILL

There is a wheel of life in me
That turns my ills away,
It grinds away the strife I see
That comes with every day.

It churns along with love and hope,
The grist within my soul.
It enables me to live and cope
With troubles that unfold.

This wheel of life I lubricate
With God's own precious words,
Which clears away all sin and hate,
The grime that oft' occurs.

I keep it turning day and night
To keep my bearings straight,
Around the axle of my life
Until my judgment date!

"THE SUBSTITUTE"

I've been writing poems and verses for several years now and the best way I can describe the effort is that they are neither too hard or too easy to accomplish what I want to say in a particular theme. However there are times when I become a total blank, so I have to make out the best I can until something comes along. The short verse "The Substitute" is an example of that.

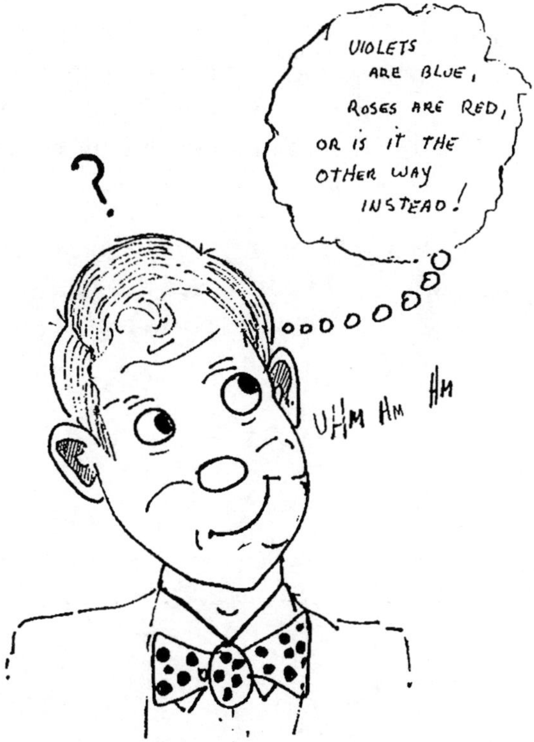
VIOLETS
ARE BLUE,
ROSES ARE RED,
OR IS IT THE
OTHER WAY
INSTEAD!
UHM HM HM

THE SUBSTITUTE

Here I stare at my notebook bare
With my pen all ready to go;
And my mind is there, but my thoughts won't bear,
And the words refuse to flow.

It's the way it is with a poet wiz
When he thinks he knows it all;
And its lines he'll miss of poetic bliss,
When he runs into this wall!

So I sit in a kink and my eyes I blink
With my tongue curled up in my cheek;
'Cause I just can't think of any thoughts to ink,
And the effort looks mighty weak.

It's awful tough to write this stuff
When the thoughts won't come my way;
So off the cuff I tried this bluff,
And I wrote this poem today!

❖❖❖❖❖❖❖❖

"ODE TO OLD RETIREES"

I suppose the only retired person I really ever knew before I came one, was my father. He was 46 years old when I was born so he was really nearing retirement at my early age. I came to view the behavior of a retiree sooner than most folks do under their circumstances.

Now my father retired in the heart of a depression when times were really hard and social security checks weren't even heard of. So he spent most of his time looking for small jobs around the neighborhood or raising garden vegetables to sell at the produce market. But he also spent a lot of time around the house and there-in lies subject matter for my following verse, "Ode To Old Retirees".

Now this verse is not intended to be written about my Dad, rather to all retirees, including myself, whom I believe encounter these circumstances revealed in "Ode To Old Retirees".

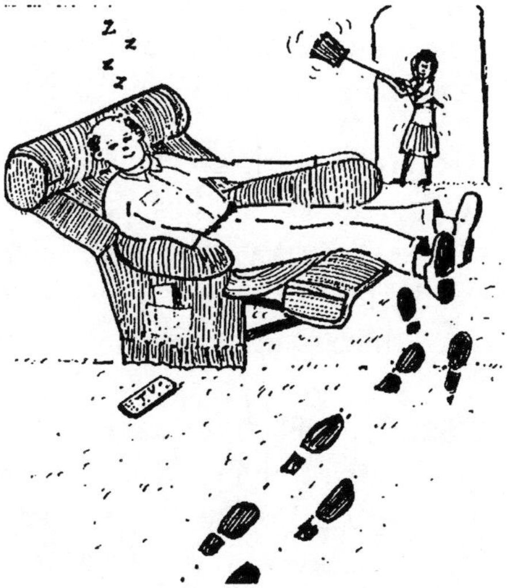

ODE TO OLD RETIREES

From out of his past
Flow memories that last,
A retiree's daily trend;
'Cause his work is blue with nothing to do,
So he pours out his past from within.

He recalls all his times
And always defines
A million things that he's done;
It now gets old as the stories are told,
That its just another re-run.

And around the house
He bothers his spouse,
Where he putters around all day.
And she scarcely can hear his comments clear
As he mutters his words away.

From the yard he got soiled
Where he piddled and toiled,
And into the kitchen he tracks
The mud on his shoes, his wife's not amused,
And her scolding she did not relax!

He has these old clothes
Which he will not dispose,
Some still carry an ancient decor;
And when he undresses, the hamper he misses,
And the clothes are strung on the floor!

And it seems all the days
That he's set in his ways,
And never does he alter his mind,
But nevertheless we all can attest
That no one is ever so kind.

But this guy can't win
If we doubt in him,
So please, try hard not to fuss,
And be good to him when patience grows thin,
'Cause someday it will happen to us.

And because after all
He has met his call,
And paid up in his life long fee;
And when he is gone we will all be alone,
When we miss this old retiree!

"SPELL OF A WATERFRONT"

For many years, my wife Bobbie, and I searched the coastlines of Virginia and North Carolina for waterfront property. Our dream was to live on the water. We would spend weekends driving many miles to answer ads about beautiful waterfront properties that turned out to be nothing more than deep ravines that contained only drain water.

Usually the real stuff was either too expensive or it had just been sold. This trend continued until 1990 when we finally found our dream spot in North Carolina on the Pungo River, Pamlico sound area. We lived there for five years at which time our waterfront hunger had been partially satisfied, and additional grandchildren had come into the fold in Virginia, so our thoughts turned home again to Virginia.

The following verse, "Spell of A Waterfront", accurately describes my feelings about it.

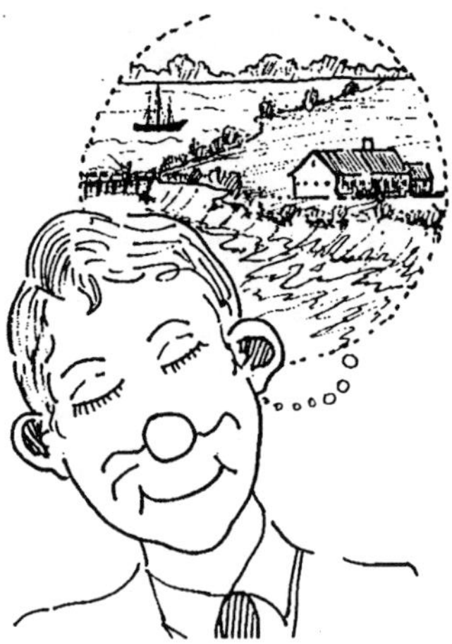

SPELL OF A WATERFRONT

I sought waterfront and I got it;
I searched for many a day,
Not once did I say quit
'Til I found it at Crabtree Bay.

I love that place on the water
Where I could go boating or fish,
But five years and a quarter
Our children we came to miss.

So we came back to "ole Virginny";
A duty is here now to fill,
But I still love my waterfront plenty,
And I plan to go back-and I will.

I think of that beauty down yonder
Where our lives were sparkled and
sweet;
Where crabs are measured a wonder
When caught there at Mattamuskeet.

Where I could go netting for minnows
From the bank along by the bay--
Or catch on my line a few winners
To make it a perfect day--

Or I could just sit there in leisure
And enjoy its sea water air;
Where quietness of inner peace pleasure
Came into my soul to bear.

Now, I've returned to the busy
Street traffic and crowds at the mall,
Outdoors, where all is so dizzy,
Oh, how I'm fighting it all!

Ah! But there is the sake of my
children
Which is all so worth the while;
To forsake on my course I'm willin'
To renew here an old life style,

But I'm doing it under submission
'Till all my grand kids are grown,
Then I'll renew my love mission
Down at my waterfront home.

But for now I'll hold it behind me
'Til I can return once more,
To the place I lived so sublimely
Down on the Pamlico shore!

❖❖❖❖❖❖❖❖

When I was a young man I armed myself with a 12 gauge, double barrel shot gun and went into the woods to hunt for deer, for the first time I might add.

I thought about how thrilling it would be to shoot one and I had heard how good the meat tasted so I looked forward to that. But what I remember about that hunting trip was that I lost my nerve when I had the opportunity to shoot my very first deer. I recall it being a very cold Saturday morning, just about daylight, when a huge buck deer larger than any I've ever seen in a zoo appear below the tree stand I was positioned in. He was only about 10 feet away and below me when he stopped and looked straight up my double barrels.

I have to tell you I was terrified with the thought of pulling the trigger. He must have sensed how "chicken" I was for he stood there for what seemed to be five minutes! He also appeared to have been slightly wounded from some other hunter's gun shot. So this helped me restrain myself. At any rate, he vanished into the brush as I still sat dumbfound catching a final glimpse of his white tail leaving the area.

Since that time I've hardly been able to swat a fly. But it hasn't been a total loss, for that hunting trip taught me to appreciate the woodlands, its habitants, and just the sheer joy of being in a part of God's world where I can really feel His presence. The following verses, "My One and Only Deer Hunt," "Sniffer," "Out Door Wonders," and "The Outdoors Man" explains my experience and love for the outdoors.

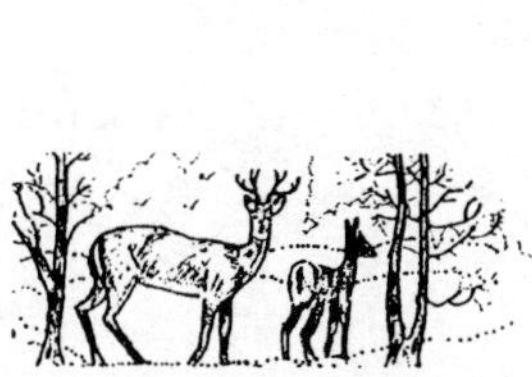

MY ONE AND ONLY DEER HUNT

I never knew the consequence
That slaying a deer would have;
But all the time I felt suspense
While going down the path.

I found a stand up in the tree
And loaded up my gun;
My hands and feet were 'bout to freeze,
My face was also numb!

It was, I knew, the coldest morn
Of many, many years,
'Cause cycles from my nose did form
And frozen were my ears.

Just sitting there all tightly drawn
With "big buck" on my mind;
I saw his doe and little fawn,
I thought, he's close behind!

I was surprised at what I saw,
My heart jumped all athrill,
My frozen blood began to thaw
On thinking of a kill!

He only stood ten feet away,
His sad eyes looked in mine.
I felt a chilling sick dismay
That traveled down my spine.

I didn't have the heart to fire,
So I just sat and stared,
For I just gained a new desire
To let this deer be spared

I still don't know the consequence
Of having shot a deer,
But now I feel much better since
I quit the sport that year!

❖❖❖❖❖❖❖❖

SNIFFER

He came one day in dreadful cold
With snow drifts all around;
The winter storm had taken toll
On this small beagle hound.

Upon my back-way stoop he lay,
No whimper could I hear,
For this young pup who went astray,
His end was clearly near.

I picked him up and took him in,
The only thing to do.
He looked so weak and deathly thin,
I thought that he was through.

His tiny sides, there was no doubt,
Was starved from lack of food,
His little ribs, they just poked out,
He did not seem to move.

His little body limp as silk
I placed there on a cot,
And with a cup of warm whole milk
I nursed him every drop.

And then I saw his little tail
Go twitching all around,
Then came the best part of this tale,
A new home he had found!

From there on out without a doubt,
This pup began to sprint,
And grow and sprout 'til he got stout
Then to the woods he went!

I've never seen a nose so keen,
He'd sniff out every log.
He was a rabbit chasing thing,
He was a "sniffing dog!"

Into the past I look with pride
At one I knew would differ.
This one great prize that almost died,
My beagle hound named "Sniffer."

❖❖❖❖❖❖❖❖

OUTDOOR WONDERS

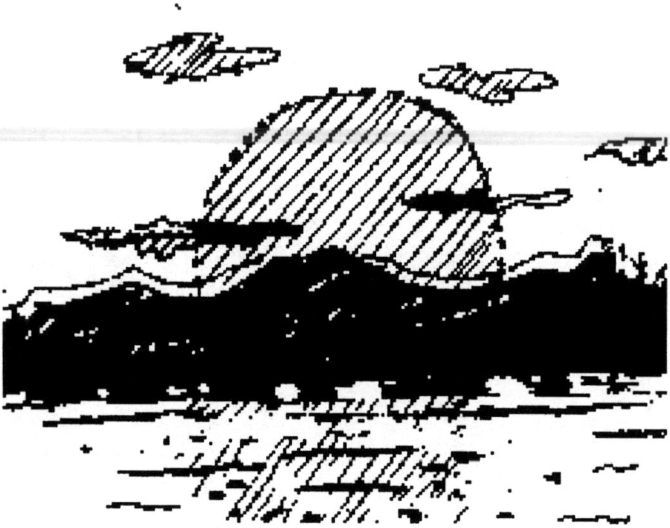

I have often stood in wonder
Upon a lofty bank,
And delved in sensuous ponder
Of the setting sun that sank;

Beyond the crusty mountain range
With its valley there below,
Along the crest of the distant plains
Or beneath a river's flow.

Beyond the bay on eastern shore
Where I've often seen it rise
In brilliant shades of color galore
That painted the entire skies.

I have also looked in reverent gaze
Into a dark moon sky,
And marveled at the many ways
God set the stars on high.

At other times, a moonlit sky,
Its gleam across the sea,
And watched the silver clouds go by
As they drifted endlessly!

Where often through my window panes
I've viewed the skies that yields
The splatter of the falling rains
Upon my window sills.

It's these bleak and rainy days I see
That brings my thoughts to bear,
To realize the ways indeed,
God shows His loving care,

And one of these, the great outdoors
Where all His creatures stay,
Is where my lonely heart explores
His masterpiece array.

Only a few of wonders true,
All gifts from God above,
Signed, delivered, for me and you
With His signature of love!

THE OUTDOORS MAN

I truly love the great outdoors,
A life I've always known;
My heart takes wings like an eagle soars
When I hear old nature's tone.

So give me the good old back hill roads,
The rolling meadow lands;
The back wood creeks where the fish abodes,
Or the beach with its golden sands,

Or spend the day on Chesapeake Bay
And dream of all that's grand;
Just wish the world would go away
And return on my command!

Or go to the busy woodlands free
Down deep in the forest glade;
Just breathe the air of ecstasy
Of the life here God has made.

Just hear the breeze in the tall pine trees,
Or listen to the whippoorwill,
Or smell the dew on the fallen leaves,
Or remains of an old wood mill.

So give me the good old outdoor life,
Not that of the busy town;
Removed away from the ills of strife,
Just buried in the joys I've found!

"EARLY EYE OPENER"

How many times can you recall driving down the highway or city street and going a little faster than the speed limit? Then in your mirror you sight a blue light from a police car and hear the shrill of his siren coming up fast behind you.

Do you recall that sick feeling in your stomach that you're about to be fined? Do you recall that great, wonderful feeling of relief when he passes you by instead? Well this is the feeling I express in my verse "Early Eye Opener."

I was only about six years old when I visited those back yards in the fall of the year for those delicious pecans, and most of the kids in those days did too. But I was naturally afraid of policemen and in this verse I explain this and how my guilty conscious was cured.

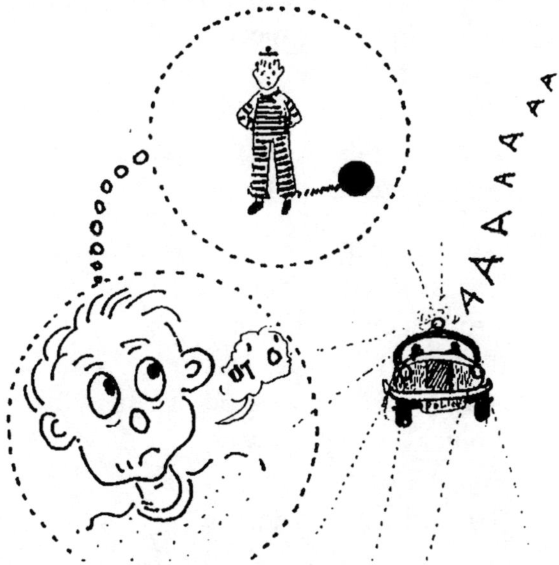

EARLY EYE OPENER

I was just a little tot in 1933
When I was scooping pecans up
Beneath a neighbor's tree.
It was to be a frightful thing,
The worst I ever saw,
For what appeared is what I feared,
Were agents of the law!

In a cloudy gust of wind and dust
They came upon the scene,
Their sirens on with deafening tone,
Their lights were on high beam!
I was so scared I never dared
To move a single limb,
For now I thought that I'd been caught
In my atrocious sin.

It's a guilty thing that fear can bring
But also brings respect,
Is when I saw the mighty law
On-rushing to inspect!
And in their flee when reaching me,
Kept going right on by
Into the house to save a spouse
Whose husband's gone awry.

Now from my fright to much delight
I learned a lesson strong.
From deep inside I now describe
There's guilt in doing wrong,
And from the pose from whence I froze
I quickly slipped away,
Age six or so I came to know
That crime does not pay!

❖❖❖❖❖❖❖❖

"BALLAD OF THE OLD COUNTRY STORE"

It doesn't matter how old one gets, we always remember some part of our childhood which we never forget, and the old country store was indeed part of mine.

I suppose one of the reasons we recall so well is we tend to tell these stories so much, it becomes a rehearsal session and the older we become, the more solid the recollection.

I guess this is the case with the "Ballad Of The Old Country Store" which accurately depicts the life and times back in those days.

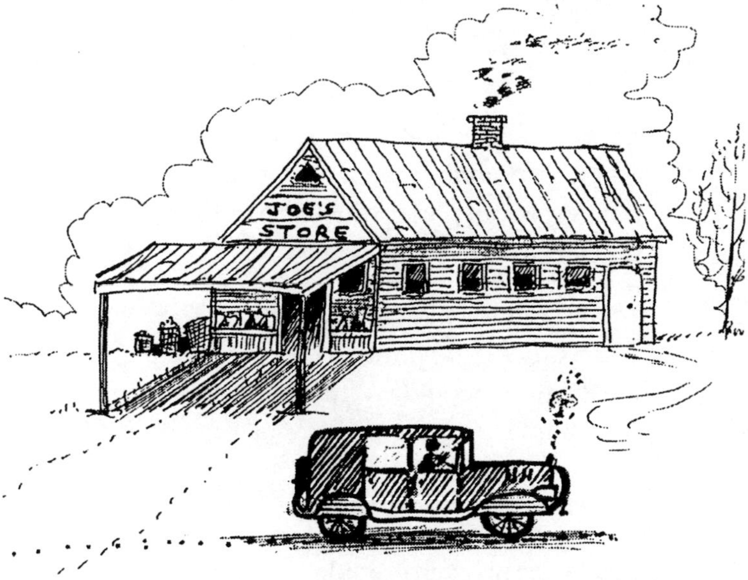

BALLAD OF THE OLD COUNTRY STORE

I finally did! I visited
My busy old home town,
Where on a lot I found my spot
Once held with much renown.

For it was here in yesteryear
That brought me total joy
Of heart-felt bliss of happiness
When I was just a boy.

In traffic's hum I came upon
Its dusty, last remains.
Now tears I fight for comes the sight
My memory entertains.

It's now folklore, this little store,
This giant that used to be,
Is now decayed but love engraved
In all its lone debris.

It was a must and it was just
A simple country store.
Where people pined way back in time
When lives were really poor.

It mattered to, and catered to
The workers at the mill,
Where folks would come in rain or sun
For all their needs to fill.

The place to be where Mom sent me
So many, many times,
And in the air were people's care,
Which showed their passion signs.

A lot of fun it was to run
The grocery errands here,
For all the folks with different strokes
Were always so sincere.

A lack of harm, oh such a warm
And friendly atmosphere,
It was uncanny just how many
Friendships bonded here.

It was a style that all would smile
When they came in the store,
The well to do, the average too,
Wide open was the door!

It was so fine for every time
I made my entry there;
Old Uncle Joe would lift and throw
Me up in to the air!

And then he'd joke, and then he'd stroke
My head of cotton white,
And with a smile that stretched a mile,
Made everything seem right!

'Twas Uncle Joe who made it go,
He owned that little place.
It was his aim to know their name
And everybodies' face,

For he was mayor elected there,
He was the people's choice.
As mayor elect he gained respect,
He was the driving force!

And council-men would come to spend
Some time at Uncle's store,
To air the cares, the town's affairs,
To represent the scores.

But after then they'd browse within,
Just hang around and hov,
Tell all their tales of spin and grin
Around the old wood stove,

Where there they sat with chaw and spat
Into the brass spittoons.
When often came a checker game,
Or hymns and gospel tunes.

With blue grass slang, the songs they sang
Came out of yesteryear,
Of tales of life about their strife
And those who fought off fear.

But this small store was something more,
To us, an entire world,
'Cause for awhile we lived a style
Before TV unfurled,

In every way on every day
It met our daily need,
Our only source of our resource
Was for our lives to feed.

Within the store, around the floor,
Were goods of many kinds:
Oats and coats, belts and pelts,
Skins from muskrats' hinds.

"Tube Rose" snuff that most folks stuff
Within their lower lip.
What once was sniff with one quick whiff,
The method is now "dip."

Tobacco "chaw" for peoples' jaw
Or 'bacco for their pipe,
To smoke in bowl, or paper roll,
Even an insect bite!

Peanuts and cups, bay rum and gum,
Cold drinks and candy bars,
Matches, crackers, cigarettes,
Grits and canning jars,

Oil for lamps, fuse plugs for amps,
Candle wax for light.
We needed these for specialties
To depend on them for sight!

Was garden seed and chicken feed,
Fat-back and salted fish,
It made no difference of your need,
This store could fill your wish.

To write a book about this nook
Would take a lot of pages,
For all the joy that was employed,
Now given to the ages.

Now, 'fore my eyes I realize
I'm looking at a heap
Of old debris enchanting me-
Will in memory keep.

❖❖❖❖❖❖❖❖

The following two poems, "To My Wife" and "Once is Enough", are my words of appreciation to my dear wife, Bobbie, for her love, understanding, and her support that has been prevalent for forty-two years.

TO MY WIFE

What can I say or do my dear
To show my love for you?
What will it take for me to make
Your dreams of joy come true?

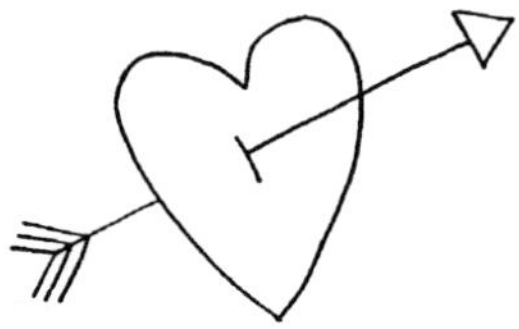

I would gather up the stars at night;
The moon with all its hue,
The silver coated clouds in sight
And give them all to you.

If I could give you all the world
'Twould be a small amount;
For all the splendor you've unfurled
Is more than I can count!

You stayed by me in thick and thin,
You're always at my side.
My love for you will never end
Like ocean's changing tide.

As sure as stars come out at night
And sunlight brings the day,
I love you now with all my might,
In my heart you'll always stay.

❖❖❖❖❖❖❖❖

ONCE IS ENOUGH

I feel so alone now that you're gone
I need you more than you know;
So please hurry back so I can retract
The words that wounded you so.

I now realize how hurt can arise
When some words are said untrue.
I made much demand which I now understand
Should not have been placed on you.

I know I was rude because of our feud,
But I promise I'll work to change;
And try not to blurt ill words that can hurt,
That start these heart-aching pains.

So return to me and then you will see
It's true I mean what I say;
For after this it's nothing but bliss,
'Cause I can't go on this way!

And we can restore our love to the core,
With this, our lives will entwine;
And I vow to you I'll always be true,
And love you with heart and mind.

"LETS DO OUR DREAMS"

We never get too old to dream. It has always been my desire that if I wanted to go somewhere or do something that would enchant my life, I would strive to make that happen.

I never thought it was easy, but it didn't hurt to plan. In the following poem, "Lets Do Our Dreams", makes my point.

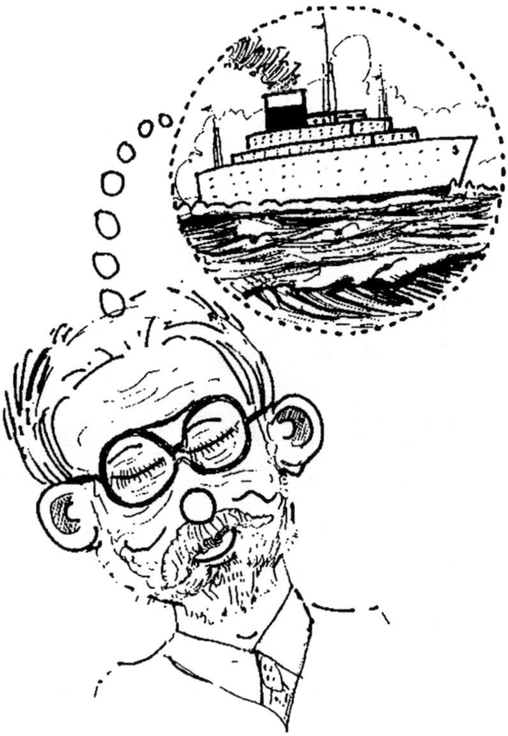

LETS DO OUR DREAM

Let's go ahead and chase our dreams, we never get too old.
Follow our star with all our means, should always be our goal.
With many more things left to do, and doing them in style,
Taking a trip to Kalamazoo would make it all worth while.
We could paint a scene of paradise of what we perceive it to be,
Or write a book on sacrifice, or one of poetry.
We could climb the highest mountain, if only in a dream;
And gather our blessings for counting to bolster our self esteem.

We could take a trip around the world and visit the castles' rare.
Let all our hopes and joys unfurl, just live our lives with flair!
To go explore the ocean's floor to look for treasures there,
Would fill me to the upmost core in finding something rare,
Another thing I haven't tried...is parachute from a plane,
Just to think that I skydived, would be a thrill sustained.
Now I realize that most of this is just a state of mind,
But that is why we all must wish and always search to find;

And If we search with all our might and dreams just won't come true,
Well, we've done our best and know that's right, yet, there's plenty more to do.
So go ahead and dream away it doesn't hurt anyone,
Could help us make it through the day, should any sorrow come.
We can still work in the garden where things of beauty grows.
Ask the Lord for pardon and mercy He bestows.
Then at the close of every day before we turn it in,
Lets ask God to show the way, when tomorrow...we start again!

❖❖❖❖❖

"ONCE UPON A CHRISTMAS"

Even today I can't really make up my mind about the concept of Santa Claus at Christmas time. It can be a sensitive issue. I think Santa in many ways has become a tool for parents to bribe or pacify their kids into a better display of behavior, but on the other hand, Santa does represent a sort of goodness that brings joy. I realize all children are not alike and can face the news in different ways when they discover there is no Santa Claus.

I guess I was a little more sensitive about it for I believed more strongly that he really did exist! I recall a genuine empty feeling when I learned the contrary at my very early age. In any event, I subsequently allowed my children to believe in "Santa" without placing too much emphasis on it, and as parents, my wife and I tried to emphasize the more important factor of all, The birth of our Lord Jesus Christ. The following poem, "Once upon a Christmas", explains my feelings on "Santa."

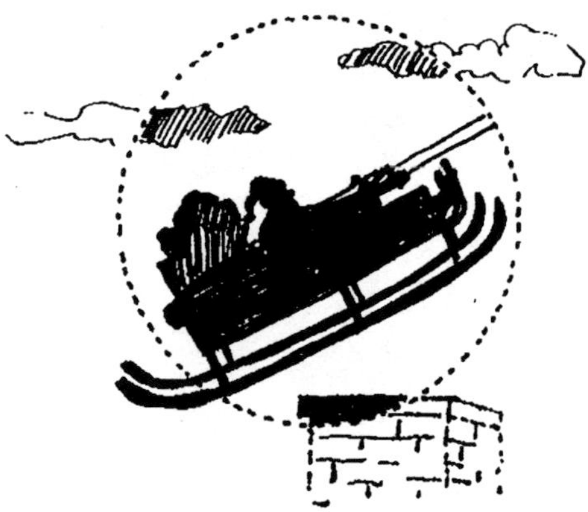

ONCE UPON A CHRISTMAS

Here is a tale I always tell
Of ages long ago.
It did dispel my "Santa spell",
And dealt a stunning blow!

I still can sight old Santa's flight
I fancied as a child,
Him, through the night with moonlight bright,
Then down our chimney aisle.

So satisfied and 'lectrified
In thoughts of Santa Claus,
I felt denied, I almost cried
For after what I saw.

For in my sleep so fast and deep,
Just dreaming dream's delight,
A noisy "beep" that made me leap
Came sounding in the night!

I had to pause to think because
I wondered about that "beep".
I did believe 'twas Santa Claus,
So I tiptoed for a peep!

With drooping jaw, through crack I saw
A very special treat.
A little car I viewed with awe,
And horn that made that "beep"!

And there that eve I do believe
My world came tumblin' down.
Instead of Santa Claus I see,
'Twas Daddy, prowling 'round!

But that new toy of Christmas joy
And pleasure on Dad's face,
Will always bring a happy ring,
For no one takes his place!

Not even dear old Santa Claus,
Whom I've really come to miss,
For yet today I stop to pause,
To think if he exists!

ANNIEBELLE

This is my tribute to Anniebelle my dedicated and loving oldest sister, who reached her eighty years on July 10, 1996.

To Anniebelle -

A toast to you dear Anniebelle
on your eightieth birthday;
you've served in life very well
with your love in every way.

We thank you for the many years
you spent and shared with us.
You did it with your thoughts and cares
and everlasting trust.

For every person in this world
a star shines bright above.
Yours is like a gleaming pearl
reflecting down God's love.

You have reached a golden age
we all would love to score.
So now we pay our homage
and wish you eighty more!

❖❖❖❖❖

TWO MORE JEWELS

My grandparents passed away before I was born, therefore I never really knew the warmth and understanding that I was told they had. It wasn't until my first grandchild that I understood this type of relationship. Before, however, I often wondered what all the excitement was about!

I also felt a little old upon that first arrival, but since then I feel that I'm getting younger as they come along. On July 29th and August 9, 1996, we had two additional grandchildren, both boys!

The following poem "Two More Jewels," illustrates our happiness.

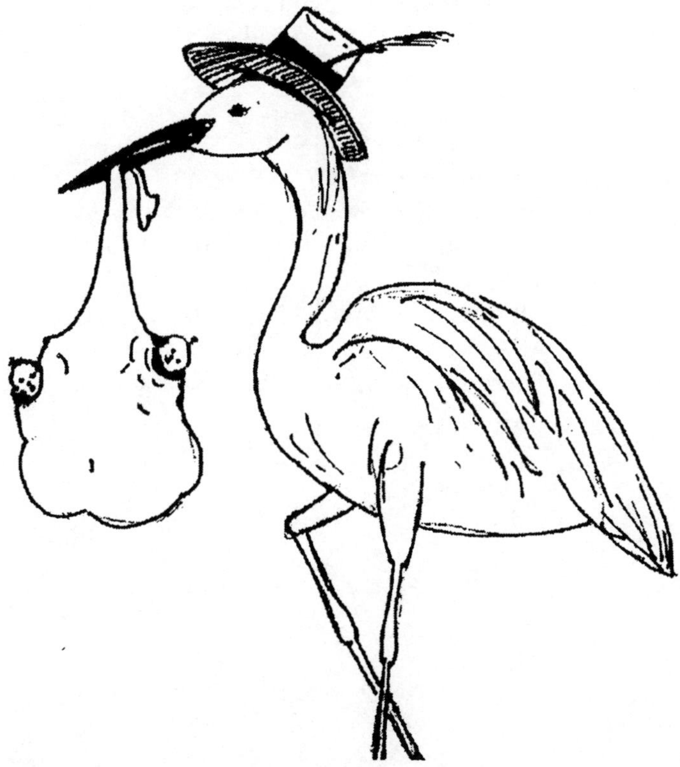

TWO MORE JEWELS

"This is the last, there'll be no more!"
Our children so had stated,
But that's a "song" we heard before,
Their "tune" is now out dated!

For comes two grandsons in the fold:
Our ego now inflates.
Just two more wonders to behold
Our hearts which now elates.

Two more jewels in our estate
Adds sparkles to our crown;
This brings the sum to number eight
To spread sweet joy around!

Two more sets of tracking feet.
("Eight will come with smacking lips")
Carpet floors to clean and sweep
From rounds of ice cream dips.

Add two more pairs of rosy cheeks,
Glowing as their joys unfurl;
We, giving what their young heart seeks.
"I wouldn't change this for the world!"

All this makes us oh so happy,
All our grand kids to adore,
These special gifts for this Grandpappy,
And Grandma for evermore.

❖❖❖❖❖

FAMILY TIES

It's hard to put in words somehow the way I really feel.
To all you dear one that I love, at times I've been a heel.
My heart has always been there; just kept it out of sight,
With ease I said the wrong thing, so tough to say it right.

But now I've come to realize to open up the door;
To say the words you want to hear, and not those from a bore!
My thoughts are always of you. I wanted things done right.
I meant no harm in stressing about life's struggling might.

It wasn't that I knew it all, that surely is a pun.
I guess I want, like everyone my place here in the sun!
So from here on out without a doubt I mean to change my ways,
To be the Dad that you deserve my everlasting days.

So here's a toast to all of you for putting up with me,
You stayed the course and saw it through, and that's my family!
Now I thank you for the good times you entered in my life.
My loves goes out to all you kids and to my darling wife!

❖❖❖❖❖

THE WOODLAND'S SUMMER BALL

Wake to the sounds of the summer morning; rise to its beckoned call.
Go while the day is here adorning, to the woodlands-free for all.
Where the forest leaves are gleaming from the drench of a morning
dew. Where dawn's sunrise comes streaming, spreading its brilliant hue.
With a trail of a magic rainbow of a yellow, red, and blue,
Casting its morning sparkling glow as the light comes passing through.

Stop! Listen to the sounds that the forest brings. The songs of the
habitants here,
the mating call that the mocking bird sings or the meadow lark that is
near.
The chatter of the chipmunk on the prowl, the crow that's atop the trees,
The "who who" of the wise old owl in the rustle of the gentle breeze.
Where squirrels all sprawl up the trees and all and a doe stands
watching her fawn;
and the lonely sound of the whippoorwill's call comes through in the
early dawn.

What a wonderful world we have out there, what a joy to hear and see!
What a fragrant smell of the morning air, what a beautiful day for me!
"Want advice?" Take mine! rise and shine, get up at the crack of dawn!
Leave your worries far behind and go where I've foregone,
to the woodlands free, for one and all, out in the early morn,
go where the action meets its call on every day that's born.
So wake up to the summer morning; rise to that action call.
Go while they're still performing at the woodland's summer ball!

❖❖❖❖❖

MY WIFE, BOBBIE

To you dear wife this Christmas Day, I express my love for you,
For all support that you display each day our whole life through.
You gave me strength when I was weak, you answered every call.
You were there when times were bleak to keep me from a fall.

You are more than just a wife to me, my friend and helper too!
You're there to look when I can't see in many things I do.
I know you're tired of hearing me ask; "where is, or have you seen?"
Without complaint you met the task with mind so sharp and keen.

I know that I should tell you more just how I love you so,
But guess it's not within my core to let my feelings go.
But I'll tell you now this special day, "I love you, my sweetheart,"
And though these words I rarely say, it's now I plan to start!

So as we live, our love will blend as we continue on,
For if you're with me to the end, I'll never feel alone.
At times a spiel made me a heel, but it didn't last, a fact,
'Cause all this time we're married still; for forty some years intact!

HUMMING BIRDS

My wife and I just love feeding the birds. Every time we've moved, and that's been many, one of the first chores we did was to install a bird feeder. They bring us so much pleasure as we watch them come and go. The Humming Bird is the most interesting of all.

Those tiny "fluttery" friends seem to have a mind all their own. What I describe in my poem, "Humming Birds," is what I saw on one of those first occurrences.

The other poem, "The Robbers," is a real life drama that goes on in the world of these creatures. What a great fascination it is to watch these animals when you have a feeder in your yard.

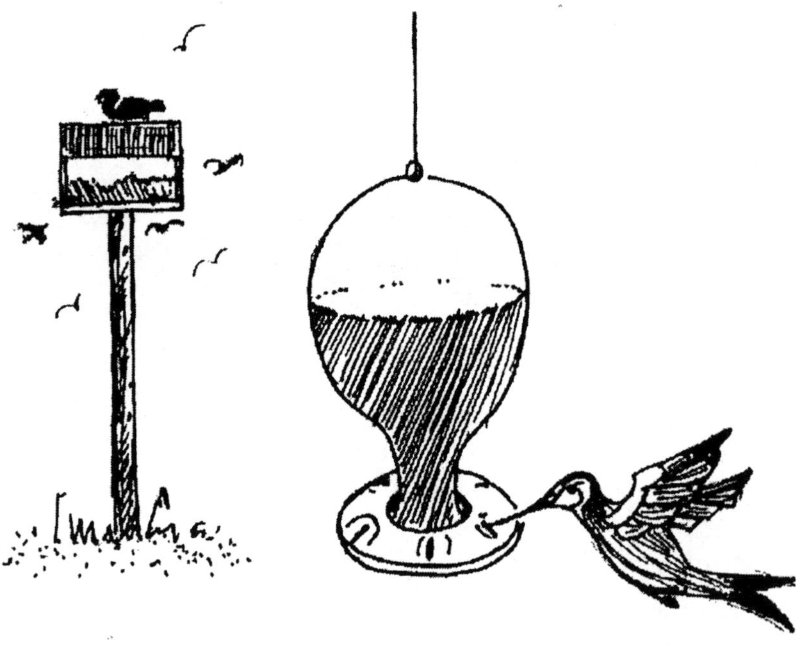

HUMMING BIRDS

From my window view I sight
a small humming bird in flight...
Towards a shrub with flowers so bright,
above, a new feeder, a special delight!
She darts past the feeder unaware
this delicious attraction was just hung there!
Her eye caught the glare of this liquid so red,
like vintage wine rare.

She stops and flutters in her retreat
and sails up to inspect this newly found treat,
And faster than the sound of her tweet,
she lands on the perch and comes to meet
this wonderful nectar, that is sweeter than sweet!
She flutters and buzzes with great delight,
Then away she went faster than light
To return again this mighty mite,
To her discovery so bright.

'Twas only a minute, lo and behold,
There came three more, they had been told
By this fluttering, feathered friend in their fold.
They remain here 'til days grow cold.
I've often wondered how they fare
Suspended there in the air.
Like a copter hovering there,
And where they go I know not where.
It's all in God's great scheme of things;
To all of us the joy it brings,
To see the humming bird come each spring
To dazzle us with their amazing wings!

❖❖❖❖❖

THE ROBBERS

I have a new bird feeder, blue, all bright and full of seed;
I'm looking through my window's view for birds to come and feed.
Here come the birds but also herds of squirrels who came to lunch;
they're loudly heard, at least two thirds are squirrels in the bunch.

They climb the post, scare off the host, devour the entire seed;
they look around and scamper down, a' gloating in their deed.
They flip and flop, jump to the top, and swing around the side;
and then they'll stop and then they'll drop and then they run and hide.

"I'll make amends fine feathered friends: I'll try to intervene.
I'll lend a hand and tie a band, and to that add a screen."
Then came the squirrels, their tails all curled in usual sneaky styles;
and feathered friends up in the limbs are chirping giggly smiles.

But soon there swoon turns into gloom while looking on the scene;
for furry friends had leaped from limbs and landed on the screen.
So there indeed goes all the seed, I'll need to think this through...
to find a lead to stop this breed, this furry, pesty crew.

So out I set a fishing net above the feeder coop;
but still they jump up from a stump into the seed they root,
and all around, the birds they frown, they peck and peep and pine;
but I am bound to find what's sound; a final stop I'll find!

Now smart and shrewd I fix a tube around the feeders prop;
twelve inches round, twelve inches down and lid that seals the top.
So now they find that when they climb there is no where to go;
they cannot move when in this tube, they just climb down below.
And now the birds, their cheers are heard, their glee is clearly sent;
'cause squirrels around eat off the ground, now everyone's content!

❖❖❖❖❖

A TOAST TO NEWPORT NEWS

Here's a great big toast to Newport News, our city here on the James;
to each and all she pays her dues, for lovers she makes her claims.
In the lap of the world she proudly sits, a giant here by the sea.
On our worldly maps she firmly fits for all the world to see.
Her railroad yards, and old shipyards have blessed us each and all,
and now it's time to show regards and keep her standing tall!

From the distant stars are better views from those who soar on high,
heroes all from Newport News, nobody will deny!
Dear "Pop" Lampkin, Julie Conn, and Donald Hyatt too,
just a few who made a bond when they were passing through.
And many times on my return on route 258
at the traffic light at Carrolton, I sight the Golden Gate...

of the bridge's span and its tower high, as high as my heart felt joy;
and a warm glow feeling crept o'er me nigh, like that of a little boy!
From across the way I could see it lay, my town of Newport News,
with a gray like haze and the sunlight's rays, showed off her brilliant hues,
and I knew right then I'd soon be there in the town I call my own,
'cause I heard its music in the air with a drone of its magic tone.

So to all the world I say to you: "You've got nothing here to lose,
so come and start you life anew in our city of Newport News."
In Newport News down by the James, may she live for ever more;
in the hearts and minds of all who claims her land from home to shore!
So here's to you old Newport News we raise our glass on high;
to city hall and all its crews that makes our city spry.
And to all the ones who paved the way so we could prosper here;
and here's a toast to every day we live in you each year!

❖❖❖❖❖

DEAR OLD HAMPTON ROADS

At first, I thought old Hampton Roads was just some "melting pot",
where people came to find abodes and work the jobs they got.
They came from far, wide and near to fill these jobs and places,
such as railroads and the shipyards here and military bases,
and it's not the same thing, I suppose, like towns they left behind,
for here in good old Hampton Roads they had new friends to find!

Well, this is how it was for me way back in '53,
and here there was good company, so here I planned to be.
I love my town from long ago down on the NC coast;
and now have dear old Hampton Roads, another place to boast!
In many ways they're both the same with water on each side,
and since they differ just in name, with both I'm filled with pride.

My memory bank holds many years of time spent near the bay.
I've seen her smiles and seen her tears while living here each day.
I've seen her mighty harbors bear the giant ships of the sea,
bringing out the pride and care of all who's here to see...,
...and how she's weathered hurricanes that romped upon her lands;
that flooded many roadway lanes and washed away her sands,
but again she stood against the storm, again she rose on high,
above, beyond majestic form, nobody will deny!

She welcomes those who come in peace and those who work with pride;
and everyone who's here at least, should with her laws abide.
From Newport News to Norfolk bound, from Suffolk, Portsmouth too,
to Chesapeake and Hampton town where dreams can all come true.
So here we are let's bear the loads and claim her for our own,
the corner stone is Hampton Roads, God bless our very home!

❖❖❖❖❖

FOUR SEASONS

I have reached a ripe old age, and I will honestly state that I have no idea which season of the year I've come to like best. In the past, like other people, I think I like the one that's presently going on, though that could easily change, should the weather decide to do so.

The important thing is they are all necessary in this life, and we have to deal with each one handed to us. My best explanation of choice is expressed in my poem, "The Four Seasons."

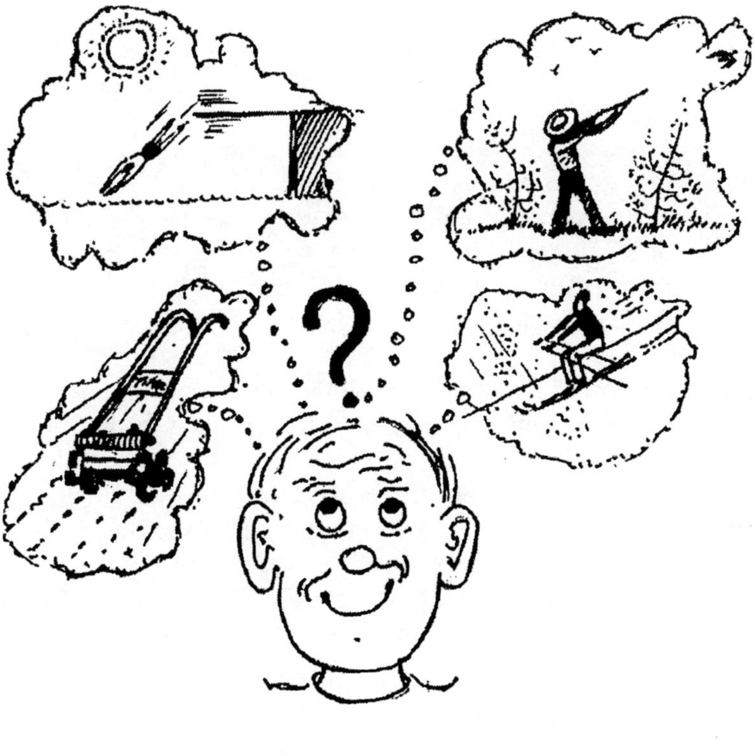

FOUR SEASONS

You ask me which season that I enjoy best?
I will answer with this reason: "none is better than the rest."
For God so molded every year into four seasons be;
and everyone is just as dear as any other three.
So in the spring comes happy things and time for all that grows;
and seeing birds on active wings, a gift that God bestows...
and purple martins come again with all their splendid soar,
coming from some far off land just as years before...
and gather in flocks upon their house with chirps of glee arriving;
no greater joy in me arouse, as that of their surviving.

So spring is special time of year when warm winds start to blow,
and natures growth, around us near, makes our adrenaline flow!
Now after spring, then summer brings vacation fun for all;
and gardens grow and over flow with vegetables grown tall...
and from my porch some summer eve when all is quiet still;
all my ills and woes take leave, at the call of the whippoorwill...
and nothing is more wonderful on any summer day;
than casting with my fishing pole in nearest lake or bay...
and also when its very hot and sweat is pouring out;
dipping in my favorite spot is ecstasy I shout!
Its just the thought of cooling off that makes the summer great,
no flu, colds with tickle cough, or worry 'bout my weight.
Yes, I love the summer days and yet, I look to fall;
for there too, are many ways that I can meet my call.

Fall is beautiful of the year when all the leaves start turning;
and all the signs of change are clear; that cold days are returning.
The trees with all their colors bright explode in red and gold;
a picture for an artist's sight, of beauty to behold!
And when these leaves fall to the ground, brings out the neighbors all;
to rake them up from all around, and relish in their fall.
Now days are brisk and nights are crisp, with cool breezes blowing,
and with the rise of morning mist, reveal the pumpkins glowing.

So now we enter winter time, Thanksgiving and Christmas comes,
when people join in holiday chime and bond with loving ones.
...and also at this special time, when yuletide season starts,
we all give thanks for all that's fine with love from all our hearts.
To enjoy our children on Christmas morn, although a hectic pace;
while in their arms, gifts adorn and pleasure spreads their face!
Which season do I like best, you ask? "They're all the same to me,
in every one, each day I bask 'cause all of them are free!"
So now I'll start another year, a fact so simple and plain,
just hold the trend I love so dear...then do it all over again.

❖❖❖❖❖

DESTINY

There is a highway in each life and each one has a bend.
They are the roads that may bring strife, or ones without contend.
We know not where our steps will lead; which route we choose to tread,
but somewhere we will "sow the seed" that grows there, hope or dread,
and somewhere down along the line we'll meet up face to face
with destiny, some point in time, where fate will take its place!

Now, only hindsight tells what knows of one's own timely goals.
The many things that life bestows, that reaches hearts and souls...,
like some dear spouse who's always near in daily "thick or thin",
and being there with loving care and when you need a friend...,
or like the small ones in their cribs all cuddled safe and sound...,
or many times they soiled their bibs when flinging food around...,
and now these children all are grown and live around the bend,
now, bringing their kids to our home, rings joy that has no end...,

and many friendships that were made, and not some, I suppose,
for all the groundwork that was laid not always bloomed a rose!
No, we never knew what other fate lay waiting down the line;
lurking there 'til judgment date, lest someone came to find!
It's all because of one right turn along life's rocky trail,
where all true fate was there to learn - success, or bound to fail!
So, "to each his own" are words that send a message without doubt;
that all these facts would not have been had we chose some other route!

❖❖❖❖❖

THE LITTLE BIG ONE

There's going to be defiance and surely be intrigue
when the Card'nals play the Giants in the Deer Park Little League;
for both these teams are winners since their records tie them up,
now they battle for the championship to take the winners cup.
There are restless hearts a'plenty as the starting time draws nigh,
and suspense is overwhelming and cheering fills the sky;
all coming from the multitudes of parents in the crowd,
a'whooping' and a' hollerin' for kids whom they are proud,
and ecstatic are these little ones who're riding on a cloud.
So from the broadcast speakers which are heard throughout the park,
come announcements of the players names...come echoes from their bark,
which brings about a roar again, again the throng goes wild,
mostly when the parents hear the name of their own child!
Now comes the magic moment when the umpire shouts to all,
"let's go, let's go, it's time to go, play ball!"
This brings about another shout as players take the field,
and the moment has arrived and excitement starts to build.
The Giants are "off and runnin'" with a man on every base
'cause the base on balls keep comin' by the Card'nal's pitching ace,
but they have a "bull pen" pitcher just in case.
Now the first out did occur with a "pop up" to LeMay,
and the second out and third was a sparklin' double play,
but the damage had been done with an extra unearned run, and the Card'nals have a look of sad dismay!
But the Card'nals roar right back with a massive hit attack, and again the game is all tied up;
and as with these two teams in every case it seems, it's mighty tough to win this cup!
So the game continues on with the errors it is prone, and both sides will score a' many run,
but it won't be very long 'til darkness comes along-and once again this one may be undone;
but they reach the final inning and the score is 10 to 10,
and the frantic coaches signal their instructions to the men.

They holler to the "bull pen" and pep talk to the bench,
they are prancing in the "dug out" for the game is tied and tense.
With a man on first and second and another one on third,
the Card'nal's coach realizes that a crisis has occurred,
so he calls on his reliever, his lanky son named Ross,
to take the mound in glory so the game won't be a loss;
but the crafty Giants are sending a pinch-hitter to the plate
to break the tie that's pending for the hour is getting late.
So from the ball park speakers that's heard in Beaconsdale, comes
announcements of relievers by the names of Ross and Will,
which brings Ross strolling to the mound, relief is spelled at last,
fast and quick is every toss, like Rolaids is for gas!
Now strides up "Pee Wee" Willy, the smallest of them all,
fifty pounds when soaking wet and standing four feet tall!
He's a giant but very tiny, but wields a mighty bat,
and the pitchers, they all fear him, whom he stares beneath his hat.
So he's called upon to substitute, he's up there in a "pinch",
he's up there willed determined to "put one o'er the fence,
but the count comes down to 3 and 2, and "outs" are also 2...and
silence stuns the multitudes when the umpire calls <u>"CURFEW"</u>!! (7:30
pm dead-line).

❖❖❖❖❖

EVERY DAY IS CHRISTMAS

It's Thursday morning,
Christmas Day in 1997.
The first thing I do is pray
to God who is in heaven.
For it's about His only Son
whose birthday is today,
a precious gift to everyone
I praise in every way,

but not just now I offer praise,
I do so all the time;
on Christmas Day or other days,
they all together bind.
Another thing it's all about
is glorify His name;
from here on earth to heaven shout
the reasons why He came!

The hustle, bustle pace is o'er,
we now can settle down,
and celebrate true reasons for
this season that we crown.
To join with our beloved ones
to share this common cause,
to understand why Christmas comes
then enjoy old Santa Claus!

BRIGHT CHRISTMAS

Now please don't take me wrong,
but when snowflakes come along,
I love to see their sparklin' glow;
but only coming down, to watch it cover ground...
and then realize we all have been snow-bound.
Way back in times of old
when winter days were cold
at Christmas time when came the falling snow,
'twas great on Christmas day
when existed horse and sleigh,

but now in modern times
It just aint so!
Then too, we're all snowed in,
In our living rooms and den,
and can't go out to get our shopping done,
but out upon the street
are those who dare to meet
in a battle of the fittest... barring none.
For all that falling stuff
has made it mighty tough,
and Christmas time has turned into a mess,
so trudging in the white
becomes an endless fight,
with everybody's spirit put to test.

So, I'll tell you what I'm dreaming,
it's a Christmas that is gleaming,
where sunny skies are pretty
blue and bright;
when all can skate and run
in usual Christmas fun,
instead of plowing
all that snow in sight!

❖❖❖❖❖

THE SONG, "BRIGHT CHRISTMAS" WITH RESPECTS TO IRVIN BERLIN AND BING CROSBY

Yes, I'm dreaming of a bright Christmas
with lots of sunshine that I sight.
May your days be sunny and sprite,
and may all your Christmases be bright.
I'm dreaming of a bright Christmas
with every Christmas tree I light,
with no sleet or slopping
to hinder us from shopping,
so all our Christmases are bright.

I'm dreaming of a bright Christmas,
just like the ones without the snow,
where the streets are missing...
the slush and slipping,
or cars and people on the go.
I'm dreaming of a bright Christmas,
one where we're out and not snow-bound;
with our friends we visit,
and everyone will wish it--,
a merry Christmas cheer to all around.

I'd be dreaming of a white Christmas,
if we had a horse and sleigh,
like those of long ago...
when there was a Christmas snow,
but in our day and time...
there is <u>No-Way!</u>

So however you may take 'em
come sunshine, rain or snow,
you can always surely make 'em right;
just spend the time aglow
for the reasons that we know,
and may all your Christmases be bright!!

❖❖❖❖❖

ANOTHER CHRISTMAS

'Tis another Christmas on its way, you feel it in the air,
it all began Thanksgiving Day with bargains everywhere.
Is there a Christmas spirit here where folks go on their sprees,
and shop around with yuletide cheer for thousand dollar trees?

or show a smile that Christmas wills to everyone around,
then show good will with dollar bills in discounts that are found?
Just blow away some hard earned pay to find the Christmas "groove",
to fill the streets with honks and beeps to get someone to move?

To beat the crowd, to shout aloud in hustle, bustle pace?
To bump and run, to beat the gun in Christmas shopping race?
It's not the silver bells that ring that makes the spirits grand,
but constant ring of "dough" folks bring, which changes hand to hand!

Now if it shows that I oppose, you're mighty right I do!
'Cause I resent the money spent to make a Christmas true!
I'll take my Christmas nice and slow, which is a better way,
small gifts to go to ones we know on Jesus Christ birthday...

...to decorate a small tree bright that came fresh from the glade,
with little things that flashes light and things the children made,
and take this special time to share, to sing, to love, to see:
that Christmas time is meant for prayer, that's what Christmas means to me!

❖❖❖❖❖

A MATTER OF TIME

I'm waiting for my ship
which hasn't yet come in;
but in my heart I know it won't be long,
for even as I pine
of this "Dream Boat" on my mind,
the echo of its steam-horn sings my song.

Now in my anxious view
as I gaze across the blue,
I see her silhouette against the sky;
where across horizon's zone
with a cargo all my own,
she's bringing home to me my "piece of pie"!

There, beyond the foam,
I glimpse her coming home...
steaming on to fill these goals of mine.
I'm caught up in a trance
and the butterflies all dance
as she speeds along across the brine.

For soon I'll ride her bow
as we sail on here and now
and brush away the ocean's spray;
and when she carries me
to my port of destiny,
"I'll be king of my domain", as winners say!

❖❖❖❖❖

THE UGLY DUCKLING

When Mom and Dad were married up way back in World War I;
they did not plan a family clan, just hankered for one son.
Times were quite depressin' then, a house and farm to run,
and Dad could use a helpin' hand that comes from siring one,
but fate would deal the players hand which dealt my folks a "straight,"
for fourteen years six girls they reared with no sons to equate,
(and time was getting late!)

My Dad had gottin' up in age and Mama, she was tired,
and if they don't get what they want,with females they'll be mired.
By then the farm had all run-down, and diapers all piled up,
and Daddy's aims had still not changed, he did not have enough!
So they "set sail" to birth a male to fulfill Daddy's aim:
to work the farm, go arm in arm, to carry on Dad's name.

So, now the year is '28 and all are filled with joy,
'cause Mom and Dad have changed the fad with bouncing baby boy!
Now, due to fate Dad had his mate, but yet dissatisfied;
'cause he wants more to tie the score, the goals is set for five.
This was an aim to start a chain; 'twas five more males they sought,
but in their try for that next guy the effort went for naught,
for in the world came one more girl which brought a screechin' halt!

So, broken is that starting link and now the idea's cold,
but, Mom and Dad, eight kids they had with one son in the fold.
Well, all in all I'm happy now, but life back then weren't free;
'cause gloom unfurled with all the girls kept gangin' up on me!!

❖❖❖❖❖

TO VIRGINIA

We sing on high our praises to
Virginia, great and strong.
Amid the leaves of dogwood trees
the cardinals sing their song.

From mountains grand to coastal sand,
there's joy in every place,
for everyone beneath her sun
is treated as one race.

From Shenandoah to Eastern Shore,
from borders south to north,
she stakes a claim in lover's name
with history that come forth;

Of presidents and stately gents
who pioneered our cause;
the native sons who were the ones
who wrote our country's laws

Oh Virginia, Oh Virginia,
may your spirit never die,
in Commonwealth our love is felt
with banners waving high.

❖❖❖❖❖

GLORY TO VIRGINIA

Virginia, Oh Virginia,
the rapture of our fate;
we dedicate both heart and soul
to our beloved state;
to commonwealth so quaintly old,
so strong and ever great!

We pledge allegiance to her name,
Virginia, true and free;
'tis here where lovers make their claim
and where they long to be,
where residents of early fame
were giants in history.

So sing our toast to old "sore back".
May spirits always bloom;
as does her flowering dogwood trees,
where cardinals croon their tune;
and in the Blue Ridge Mountain breeze
drifts blossom's sweet perfume.

Virginia now and evermore
so glorious and grand,
where folks of races live as one
in our most treasured land;
to fine a "place here in the sun",
with peace for every man.

❖❖❖❖❖

FOOD FOR THOUGHT

Here is some food for thought
that most of us were taught;
to remind ourselves each day of what we know;

that everything we eat,
whether bitter, salt or sweet...
are what we are down from our head to toe;

that every thing we drink
controls the way we think,
so be careful what we pour into a glass,

and be careful what we eat
so the people whom we meet
won't view us as a dumb and simple ass!

❖❖❖❖❖

MEMORIES

LOOKING BACK

Time seems short if I just glance back over the years to any particular event or occasion; however, sometimes I think back in sort of a sequence, one might say, and when I do that, it seems like a much longer period of time.

I enjoy looking back and reviewing the many good times that I had, and I reminisce upon them. Sometimes, when my siblings are over, we'll just wallow in the joy of recalling those memories.

As a senior citizen, I've seen the many changes that progress has brought; and while I know we can't stand in the way of progress, it adds a little sorrow or sadness to my way of thinking. "Looking Back" and "My Old Town" are two poems that exemplify these changes.

LOOKING BACK

I often ponder while in thought how progress changed our ways,
of all the differences that it brought from since my childhood days.
Like on Dad's spread of yesteryear, where yet I see him now,
trudging along in awkward veer behind a mule and plow.

Carefully working down each path as he plowed back to and fro,
running into a little wrath as he made the old mule go!
At one end was the shady end where Dad would stop the plow;
to take some time to catch his wind and wipe his sweaty brow.

And he often mumbled during that time as he lingered in the shade;
"Lord! There's got to be another kind of tool besides this blade!"
He never knew the twirling tines that came to till each row,
and never saw the big combines that reap the crops below.

And I suppose in all his dreams He'd never see the day;
that all those fancy farm machines would ever come his way.
No, those were the years of the Model "T", hard work was the only rule;
the only farm tool Dad would see... was the rear end of that mule!

❖❖❖❖❖

MY OLD HOME TOWN

'Twas loved by me, down by the sea, this little town of mine,
her name is Wilmington, NC, down on the east coast line.
Many, many years ago, I left my old homestead,
when population high and low - just thirty thousand head!
My little town of Wilmington, port city near Wrightsville Beach,
where all could fish, swim or sun and easy there to reach.

I spent my youth in Wilmington and roamed her sandy hills,
found my "place there in the sun", and there I had my thrills.
A quaint old place of yesteryear when streets were cobbled stone,
a friendly, happy atmosphere, I never felt alone.
The old oak trees with moss abound just drooped in strange decor,
brought out beauty all around and showed off her folklore.
Hanover High, the only one, mid schools, Isaac Bear,
Winter Park and Tileston School, and Bradleys Creek was there,
but that was all so long ago with many changes made,
to name them all would be too tall, too many plans were laid!

Sometimes I go to my hometown,a place I once called mine,
and always ride and look around to see what I can find;
and what I see amazes me how such a tiny place
could reach a height of misery in such a torrid pace.
I looked to find my grade school ground, our house on Lingo Lane,
but understand they're not around is info. that I gain,
that it's six lanes of torture pains called Oleander Drive.
I'll never see my home again where all those autos' thrive,
and all the rest, what once was best, has left that peaceful scene,
and gone into some kind of test to out do each machine.

And when I go I fight the flow of mobiles everywhere,
I fight each red light's constant glow, I breathe exhausting air,
I hold my speech and try to reach some kind of self control,
while going into Wrightsville Beach, and coming back still whole!
So once I'm there, I stop to stare, to gaze at all the change.
What once was much a usual flair, it all now seems so strange.
'Cause once there was an inlet sound, oh my! how it did hurt,
for when I looked there all around, 'twas all filled up with dirt!

To think this place that brought me smiles is now a sub-divide,
of condo homes for miles and miles-"Big bucks they could not hide!"
...but in my sighs I realize that nothing stays the same,
that when we lose a precious prize,it's progress we must blame!
Progress has its place on earth, but here it came to kill--
it robbed me of my inner mirth, it stole away my will,
it brings me to my very knees, it makes me want to cry,
but if I'm harsh, excuse me please for comments that are wry.
So when I leave I won't bereave, I'll just remember when:
There was a town down by the sea when all was quiet back then....
So life goes on I must not frown, I'll try hard not to see...
all the strain that came to hound my old town by the sea!

❖❖❖❖❖

RED'S PIER

The day I arrived in Newport News, back in 1947, I discovered Red's Pier. I had hitch-hiked my way from Wilmington, NC, as a teenager looking for a job.

After leaving the old, rickety James River Bridge, my ride pulled into the Red's Pier area. Since members of my family were residing in Ferguson Park, a stone's throw from Red's Pier, this was my final stop; and I fell in love with the place. For many years I enjoyed a warm and friendly relationship with all I met there.

Fishing became a way of life for me and many folks around there back when croakers ran 2 to 3 pounds. To this day I'm surprised that so many young people know about this legendary spot. With great fondness, I express my tribute to Red's Pier."

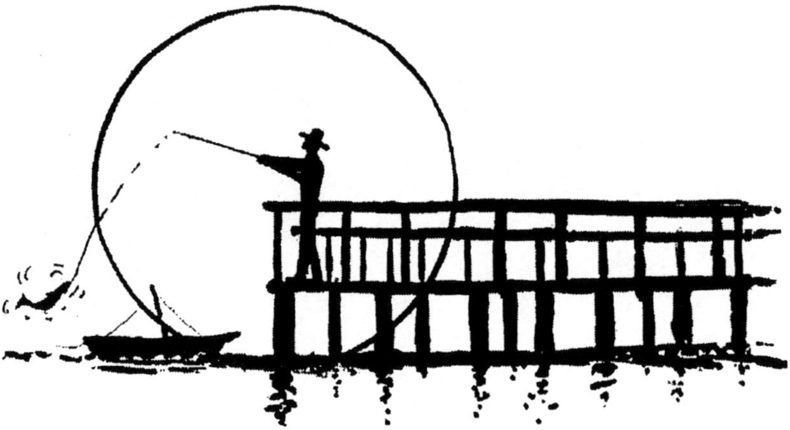

RED'S PIER

Near Huntington Park, an old land mark, and just beyond its flank;
lay a strip of land, a beach of sand, below James River's bank.
From out atop that river lot stood an aging wooden pier,
which came to be favorite spot for people far and near.
There's not a day I pass that way that memories don't appear;
of thoughts of youth and yesterday returns me to Red's Pier.
The river James, this pier it claims, where all could fish or tan,
and far across its waters came a view of the bridge's span.

Where sea gulls shrill, and anglers thrill with sounds from wind and waves,
all within my heart instill the joys that memory saves.
Where time to spend a daily trend, to meet upon Red's Pier;
no better place to find a friend or lose your woes and fear.
There is no clone left in stone, no banner flown in view...
only thoughts of it alone marks this place I knew.
A special time now comes to mind, and with it, pleasures bring,
for it was here at Red's Pier I gave my love her ring.

Since fifty-five our love still thrives, and we sometime shed a tear,
for a lasting memory in our lives of our engagement here.
And where we parked, loud speakers barked Red Crossley's firm demands.
He was heard from dawn to dark calling to his hired hands.
Yet, still I hear Red's shouts so clear that comes from long ago;
"Donnie, Frankie, come out here and get these boats in tow!"
"And fill the bin with ice gone thin and with the box unlock;
and get some bait for those who wait out on the landing dock!"

"Bring out a pail and with it bail the water from skiffs about,
and slack the ropes on the larger boats before the tide goes out."
Through the air these echoes blare with glee from kids at play,
all these things that seemed to care has long since died away.
But in my heart joy feelings start, and in my eyes, a tear,
for I know I'll never part from my memories of Red's Pier.

❖❖❖❖❖

RAILROAD MAN

About two weeks after our marriage, Bobbie, my wife, started her nursing career, and I landed a permanent job with the Chesapeake & Ohio Railroad, now known as the CSX System. Most of the next thirty-three years would be the most gratifying times of my life. In 1955, the railroad was in an explosion of activity on the Peninsula and Newport News, Virginia. The fall-out from the tremendous blast came to affect the lives of many people.

As a brakeman, I was fortunate to be a part of that huge undertaking and I gained many unforgettable memories. Now long since retired, it seems like a dream that never really existed.

The post office had nothing on us. Around the clock, in every conceivable kind of weather, twenty to thirty crews would maneuver thousands of rail cars on an hourly basis, in a very small railroad yard. All of these movements required special knowledge on skill and safety. Countless hours of braking, and many miles of walking and handling this equipment contributed to my thirty-year memory chest. There came a decline in the seventies, and a slow leak developed until the bottom drained out in the mid eighties. After the dust had settled, the boom was gone. It would be too large a task to cite or describe all the pleasurable times that took place here, but I have written a couple of poems, "Railroad Man" and "With Every Passing Train," that may be of interest to others.

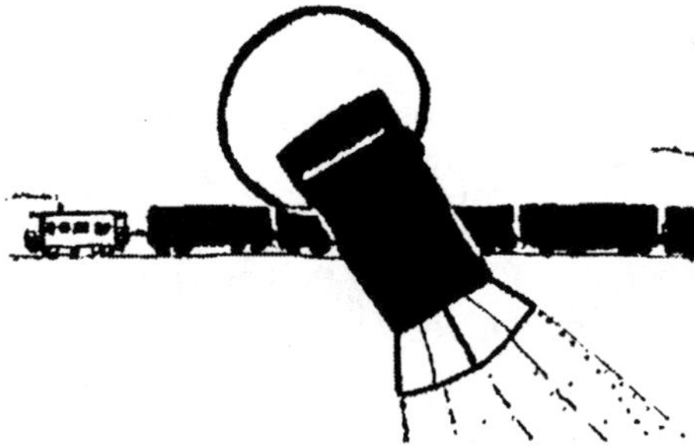

RAILROAD MAN

Once upon a time in 1955 I land a job with C&O,
which filled me with great pride! There were a lot of things to know--
but best job I could find, and came to me when I was free and only 29.
I spent three years and 30 more on railroad cars and ties;
'Twas on the yard at Newport News where all my memory lies.
Tales have come and tales have gone, I'll try to spin a few;
to cite them all would be too tall, too many to review.
So once upon a stormy night, with many more to come;
I got a call from Jimmy Dale to work on number one.
He told me that he needed me, none else would take the call;
I pled and begged and alibied, I thought about the squall!
But Dale had ways of making you say: "OK, I'll do it for you."
He said, "You'll be all right if you go tonight, they plan on working you through."
Red eyed and worn I bore the storm to hump one train on site,
but you would know two came in slow, so we stopped for lunch that night!

There was this pier called C; which had it's yard you see;
we ran all night with all our might, just like a busy bee!
We switched in a race 'til blue in the face to place the cars at C!
Next to pier C was pier B which was just as full as C.
We switched all night without delight, 'cause we stopped for lunch at three. Another pier called 8, we always got there late!
It's time to go home, a car float to come on, but we always had to wait.
We would brake in the rain, sleet, or snow, the post office had nothing on us;
we would melt in the sun, eat lunch on the run, and do it in mush and slush!
We marked up on a job called Hump; where everyone sat on his rump,
until such time the yardie would chime; "Let's go, get at em, line up!!"
The train had been bled, the engine behind, everything ready to go;
we filed out in order to mount the cars as they started to flow.
We rode with delight tied brakes with might, and went into tracks too tight;
where cars would bunch with a tremendous crunch, leaving coals dust in our sight!

The best choice of the men? Of course, the old "coal bin."
You could watch TV and lounge with a grin, til only when "Trainie" walked in!
What was the choice of the hoard? "The brakeman's extra board" and 'twas on this list to be;
you could take any call or not work at all, just live the life of Riley.

We wore the keys to fit the locks; we wore the boots for walking on rocks;
swung lanterns at night to see the light; and rode atop cars to keep engine in sight.
We humped all the trains, bled brakes that they bore;coupled hoses 'til our hands were sore!
In just one shift we walked for miles ,yes, did it often with smiles and styles.
This Newport News yard is no longer the same; has weathered the years, has only its name.
Memories galore of men alive, those that came around '55.
30 crews called in those busy days, but now there are only 3;
most of the yard has disappeared--- from here to eternity.
Much more can be said about this past; mountains of memories of a task that last.
I could write on forever, but you get the jest; the time of my life, --the very best!
As I think back today as much as I can; 'Twas a hell of a life for this railroad man!

❖❖❖❖❖

WITH EVERY PASSING TRAIN

They come from years of toiling in nights of cold and rain;
through days when heat was boiling, in times of stress and strain.
From the restless winds of winter when the countless snow storms blow,
to the beautiful days that enter, are the memories that I stow;
but many tales are spinning, I'll only cite a few;
too many things beginning and ending to review.
When in fifty-five it started, I found the C&O,
until the time I parted, my life was changed, I know!

'Cause I loved those years of treading up the paths beside the track,
coupling air hoses, sweating, and relaying the signals back.
In many times of weather, in snow drifts white and deep,
we got those trains together for schedules they must keep.
Ah, the sound of engines roaring, and ramble of rolling steel,
seeing clouds of coal dust soaring as we drove 'em to the hill!

Yet, I hear those hand brakes winding, and air brakes that were spilled;
what was once a massive grinding is now so deathly stilled.
Where on the ladders climbing, and with the grab irons hold,
comes back the thoughts reminding of days gone by of old!
Now this railroad yard has dwindled to crews of only three,
and the thirty crews once kindled is lost to eternity!

How could this work explosion with much tremendous worth,
decline with mass erosion so quickly from the earth?
This question that I'm posing, "It's progress" experts claim,
but by bits our railroads closing with every passing train,
and in my heart forever when I look upon the past,
I know my once endeavor will in my bosom last.
This rumblin' tune I'm hearing, a song with its refrain;
the music is so endearing with every passing train!

❖❖❖❖❖

MEMORIES OF A COUNTRY FARM

What wonderful and exciting times I enjoyed when I was just a boy, growing up in the environment of our homesite in North Carolina. I learned early how to milk a cow, work with tobacco crops, husk corn, etc. I never knew the pleasures of golf or any of the modern electronic games of today. Back then, in the mid-thirties, farming was not a business as it subsequently came to be. Rather, it was a way of life, to survive, "to live off the land" so to speak. At any rate, I enjoyed the chores assigned to me, and the memories are still strong. This poem, "Memories Of A Country Farm," accurately depicts the lifestyle existing then.

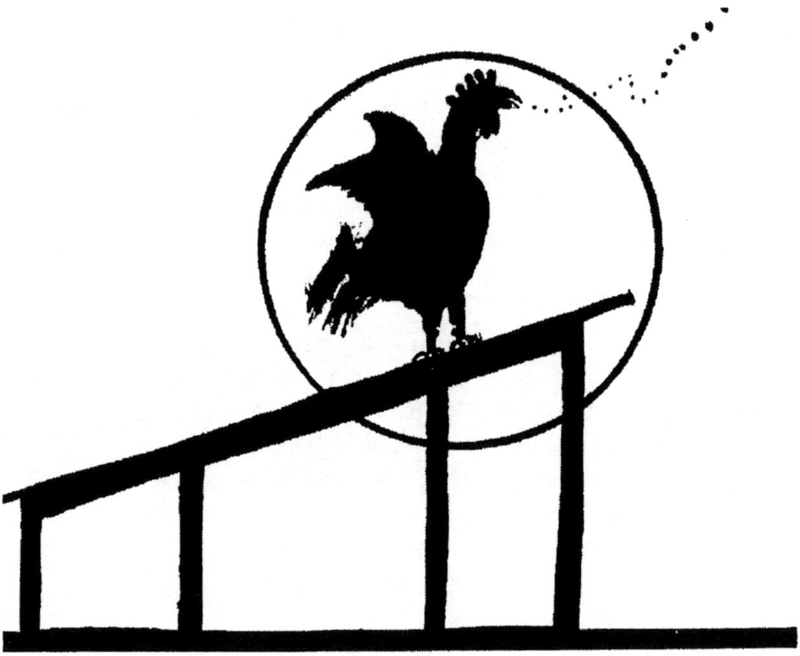

MEMORIES OF A COUNTRY FARM

When I feel low in a pensive way and the world seems so forlorn;
my thoughts all stray to an early day, to place where I was born.
In an old frame house on a country farm mid corn and tobacco crops,
where the rooster's crow was our alarm to rise and tend those spots....
and as we rose each early morn, the aroma was everywhere....
of the sweet smell of that old farm as its presence filled the air.
When the rooster stood on the chicken's coop, making his presence known;
the hens would cackle like they had croop, when heard his early tone!
Where I learned how to milk a cow, by squirting it in a pail,
to avoid her twitching I made a vow, "Stay clear of her switching tail!"
Now I think of nights back on that farm when neighbors all came to hum...
around the fire at our 'bacco barn as fiddles and banjos strum...
and pa would set a rag on fire to smoke the "skeeters" away...and all
would sing and never tire, sometimes to "break of day."
And many nights, in awe I gazed at skies with countless stars,
and all us kids would look amazed in guessing which was mars...
and dark of night was sparked by light... from lightning' bugs about.
Just one small sight, but showed God's might... He didn't leave anything out!
And from the woods late in the day, when all was soft and still,
you could hear it in a lonesome way, the call of the whippoorwill.
I'll always speak of our old brick well, a mainstay in our lives,
without a bail with wooden pail, no farm life there survives!
And mama would ring a dinner-time bell that carried way--cross the field,
and we would wash by that deep well-- on way to our noonday meal...
...and cooking aroma would drift, like haze, through woods and over the dell...
and farmers noses, like deer would raise, to breathe that gorgeous smell.
And meals prepared were carefully cared, 'cause mama left nothing out!
There were collard greens, and corn and beans and sweet potatoes pared;
ham with grits and brussel spout, (was all our stomachs could bear!) Now
those good days of long ago just fills my memories store,
Now I'm aged and gettin' slow, I cherish them all the more.
So I'll hold in my memory for now and forever,those days that filled with charm...
that when I become lonely, my first endeavor...is recall our country farm!

❖❖❖❖❖

OUR OLD COUNTRY CHURCH

There were in my life many special times and events that continue to live in my memory. On of those came when I was very young. My Mom and Dad were members of a Baptist church that held their meetings every Sunday, but they met at different locations in the state of North Carolina.

None were very far apart; however, it required some travel, and when we went to church it usually took all day. It may be unusual for other churches to present more than one preacher or minister, however, at this church's services there would be no less than five preachers who would take their turn at the pulpit.

These men were usually farmers, so they did not charge for services, as if hired by a congregation. However, they were always grateful in accepting any donation from the members. After church services, every one would branch out to some local member's home for dinner. After these meals, the folks would sit around and talk. Someone would pull out a guitar or banjo and all would join in with song. Some, depending upon their travel, might spend the night. There was always plenty of room. The memory of that activity inspired the poem, "Our Old Country Church. "

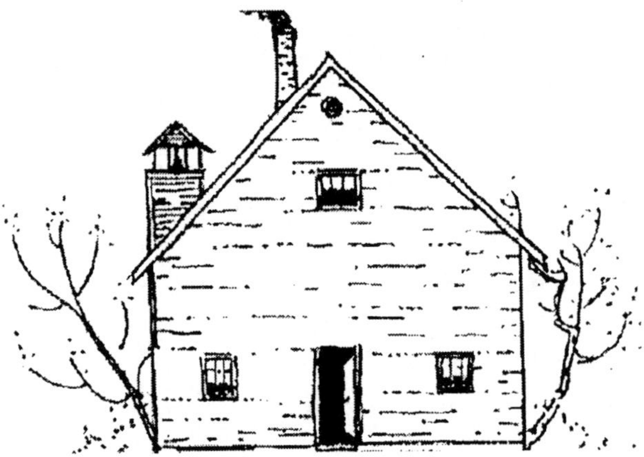

OUR OLD COUNTRY CHURCH

On a recent stay last Sunday at a place called "Maple Hill,"
I looked around and made my way to a church I yearn for still.
I went to see what used to be the dearest spot on earth,
where Mom and Dad, along brought me to enjoy all its worth.
Now, it's mostly leaning, but all its meaning comes back in memories joy,
I found myself in thoughts daydreaming of then when I'm a boy!

I saw the steeple where all the people once loved those chime bells ringing,
they would come in Sundays sequel, and join in hymn book singing.
That little church, to see it hurts, is now an old land mark;
out back I found in lonely search, the grave yard, old and stark!
And through this church grows one white birch, a measure of time long gone.
Among those limbs birds come to perch when summer days are done.

This church was bright when painted white, has withered to lime stone gray,
through wear to tear the roof shows light from skies of night and day.
The old chimney stands in crooked spands, amid the rubble there;
and wild oak vines up sides they ran through cracks of every layer.
As I looked upon that spot I'm fond my memories went inside,
where everyone met in solid bond, to pray, to cry, abide.

The people there were kind and fair, and hugged upon their greeting.
They washed each others feet with care in each third Sunday's meeting.
And when I went to church and spent almost an entire day;
five preachers to the pulpit went with sermons their own way.
They all spoke long 'bout the Bible strong, and some folks rose in shame,
confessed their sins and all their wrong to answer in God's name!

There came a time a heart did shine, and one man heard his call,
when asked to come and with God bind, he commenced to cry and bawl!
He left his seat still trembling yet, and stumbled to the pulpit stand,
and with the preacher in a hug they met, took a burden from this man.

Now I was told he was in from the cold and knew no Bible verse,
but after born again, behold! preached hell from the devil's curse!
And many a day he preached away and not once did he look;
as the Bible lay on the shelf to stay, but his words came from that book.

Now I defy any normal guy to explain that mystery;
How that man could preach on high without prior knowledge be.
And I can recall my mother's shawl, a Christmas gift from me,
and I remember some tear drops fall when she looked and smiled at me.
And I remember my Dad so limber, when called upon in leading
the congregation and each member, in song and Bible reading.

And they sang out in glorifull shout, they hugged, they sighed and cried,
we loved this church with hearts so stout, a fulfillment was supplied.
This church was small now gone and all, but its memory will stay forever
in minds of those who can recall, of God's once great endeavor!

❖❖❖❖❖

OLD FRIENDS

I've been away from my hometown, Wilmington, NC, since 1952. I graduated from high school in 1948, so I had another four years to know the people I went to school with before my departure. Since that time, I've tried to contact some of my closest friends but mostly to no avail. I'm very fond and proud of those particular days, and often recall the events that took place then. The following poem, "Old Friends," pretty well describes my feelings.

Oh how I miss my early years
And friends I loved so well;
They all have gone their separate ways,
Just where, it's hard to tell.

Where are they now, my old dear friends,
The ones that shared my life?.
It can't be said just where they are
With times so filled with strife.

I guess some joined the great beyond,
While others just grew old;
But I recall from early youth,
Fond memories to behold!

All sweet memories of pals back then,
Oh how they linger still;
For in those days there were no fears,
Just happy times to fill.

There was school and work, also play,
Where many hours were spent,
But now I'm gray, and so are they,
I wonder where they went!

❖❖❖❖❖

MOM AND DAD

If I should start to say or write all the things about my Mom and Dad that express my feelings, I wouldn't have enough time left on this earth to do so. As long as I hold the memories and the love I have for them in my heart, that will be sufficient.

They both lived to be well over 90 years old, and in their early life and marriage, it wasn't easy. They coped with the great depression and raised eight children during that time. If people ever tried to live by the Golden Rule, it was them. They deserve every bit of God's blessing. Only a small part of my sentiment is shown in "Mom and Dad."

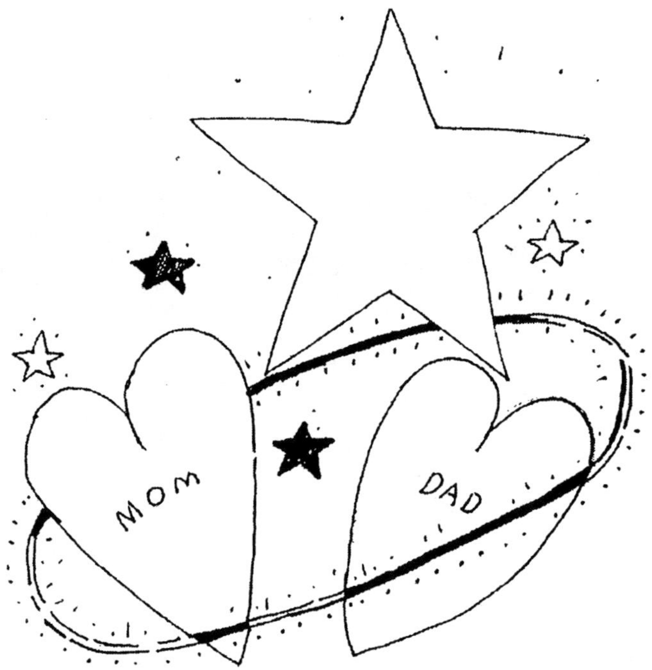

MOM AND DAD

Oh how I miss my Mom and Dad, they're in a better land;
They lived for God with all they had, and now they hold His hand.
But they had ways, as we all do, and now I understand;
They had to raise a stubborn crew, eight kids to reprimand!
I really wish that they were back so they could hear me say;
The loving words I kept intact before they went away.
It wasn't that I didn't care, respect I did apply;
My words of love were hard to spare 'cause I was mighty shy.

I never could express that word called love -- we all lay claim,
No better parents did I deserve, no better friendships came.
When other parents scream and scold, they'll suffer more than kids,
And good results will not unfold of what their sanction bids;
But Mom and Dad were both in tune, and had the best of styles;
Instead of fuss and growl and fume, they spanked us kids with smiles!
They did what they had in mind; their chore was not in vain;
The hurt was planned for our behind, not them to bear the pain!

When they spoke firm with grinning smile, it came quite clear to me;
"To spare the rod and spoil the child," was not their "cup of tea!"
Those times are gone and thoughts I store adds much to my regret;
That I didn't say "I love you" more before their time was met.
But when I pray, I tell them, as I say it to the Lord
For I know that they have joined him and all will hear my word.
And now I say to you, "Please Heed; don't throw your chance away,
But tell your Mom and Dad with speed: "You love them every day!"

HANDS OF TIME

How many families on this earth own Grandfather clocks, either store bought or handed down by their parents? I have no idea or guess, about the many poems that have been written about them. I do know about mine, which is now over 100 years old. The poem, "Hands Of Time," accurately depicts the story behind this clock.

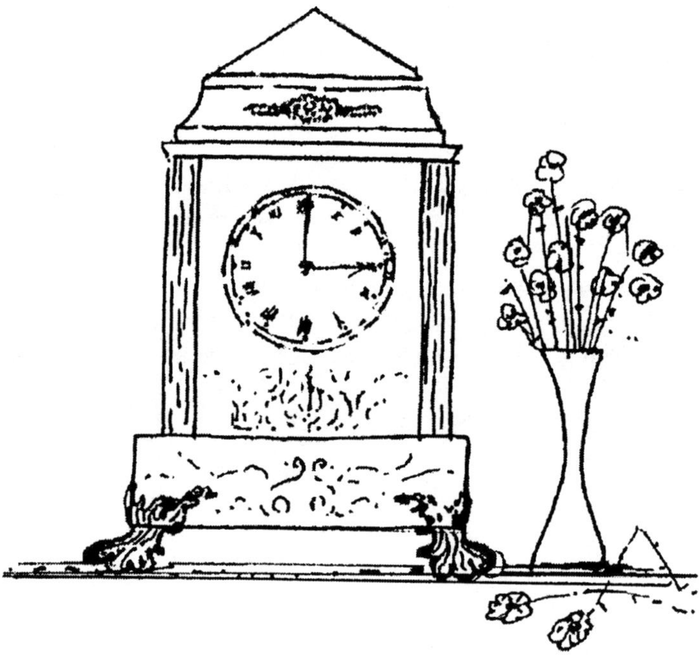

HANDS OF TIME

I keep upon my mantel shelf an old grandfathers clock;
reminds me daily of its wealth with every tick and tock!
Given to me by my old Dad the day before he died;
most priceless thing I ever had in which I take much pride.
My Daddy loved that antique clock he found in early life;
by trading off a wooden crock and one dull carving knife,

and proud he was about that deal he often spoke with pride;
how he made a bargain steal with smile he could not hide!
And from my youth comes thoughts of when-each night at
our bedtime,
Dad would wind the hands at ten and bell that rang the chime,
but now I think I understand the symbol in his mind;
for Dad, like any other man, was keeping track his time.

This same old clock that passed his time is passing mine away;
the same old tick, tock, and chime will be my child's some day.
And if he or she will come to see the meaning of its worth;
their measurement of time will be their joy while here on earth.
For more than just a clock I see; it shows me every day,
of my most treasured memory, of Dad, who's long away.

❖❖❖❖❖

ON THE MOVE AGAIN

Here we go on the move again, this is the umpteenth time;
The same old song and its refrain, and my wife is in a bind!
It all began in '55 upon our wedding date, we both were young and "so
Alive" and patience could not wait.
Our honeymoon we won't forget for travel wasn't far,
And that's because of woes we met with an old chrysler car;
Which started to cast a steamy blast from its radiator tank,
And every puff of smoke it passed, I cussed that blanky-de-blank!
But we aimed to reach our bedding spot, but not before we tried
To trade the thing at some used lot... but dealers there denied.
So we struggled around but finally found repairs on that old tank,
Only to find the brakes unsound, and motor wouldn't crank!

But after a while we start to smile, for things turned out alright,
For after trial and many a mile... we made it to bed that night!
Then on back to Newport News next day with repetition,
And this (x!Qx!?) car, black smoke it spews, is bound for demolition!
Now our first house was paid by rent for only just a while;
And here some married life was spent, where work was just a mile.
While there we lived our simple lives, but then we moved once more...
To our first home...we built a prize, with all its joys in store...
But lo and behold, as it turned out, (I guess I should have known,)
The job I had kept me in doubt, so we sold that pretty home.

Now back to Stuart Gardens we went, this time without much glee,
'Cause first of married life was spent at this same old spot, you see!
But it was fate for us to wait for things brought interest yet,
'Cause in our case we changed our base, and moved again you bet,
To our brick home we also built on huge York County lot,
But to the hilt our spirits wilt... and gone was that good spot.
So then we moved to Beconsdale and lived a modest style,
But twenty years, and without fail, the jet planes drove me wild.
This forced us out to Suffolk land, wide open spaces there;
But City Hall made much demand, was more than we could bear.

We built this home, one huge "Cape Cod," and thought we're satisfied -
We landscaped yards and worked the sod..., but this dream also died.
We lived so long and longed so strong for waterfront property,
And after years it came along --, Belhaven filled our glee.

Now five years here...Its now a fact,
Our waterfront dream is o'er, for all our moving to and back--
Has come to be one more--, just one more trip for us to roam--
To reach full circles's lane -- to Newport News, our final home...;
And there, we shall remain!

❖❖❖❖❖

CRABTREE BAY

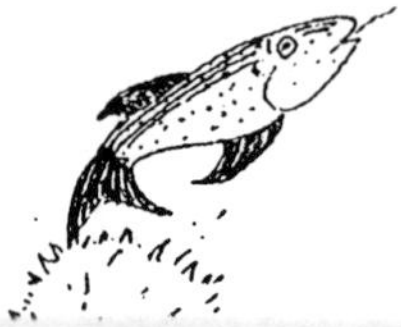

Once upon a long time dream which we
fulfilled one day;
it was to us to be supreme, a home on
Crabtree Bay!
It is a place there to behold with all the beauty
there;
where squirrels all roam and deer patrol, and
there are also bear.

And many birds and geese abound, and many otters play;
with Pungo River all around we fish our life away.
And when I look across the way, especially in the West,
the sunsets there at Crabtree Bay are surely at their best.

The colors there are most divine, the reds, the blue and gray,
nothing meets the eye more fine than sight of Crabtree Bay!
On moonlit nights the water shines, it makes you feel serene...
in Crabtree Bay where we opine about this place we dream.

We worked this spot and cleared the lot, we planted shrubs and trees,
we spent our time in fixing up and also raking leaves.
Our time lived here is almost gone, reluctantly we say;
our plan is now to interrupt our life at Crabtree Bay.

We must be moving on because destiny called us back.
We go with slow and painful pause to lay another track.
Our love, our thoughts will always beam, forever they will stay
in our hearts and every dream of life at Crabtree Bay!

❖❖❖❖❖

GONE BUT NOT FORGOTTEN

I often wonder if other people have some element of time, or something in their lives that controlled them in some way - for example a fad, a game, or some type of exercise they were involved in, then, later in their lives look back on it in an nostalgic way. This happened to me in many ways, but the following three poems depict the most important and rewarding times of my life.

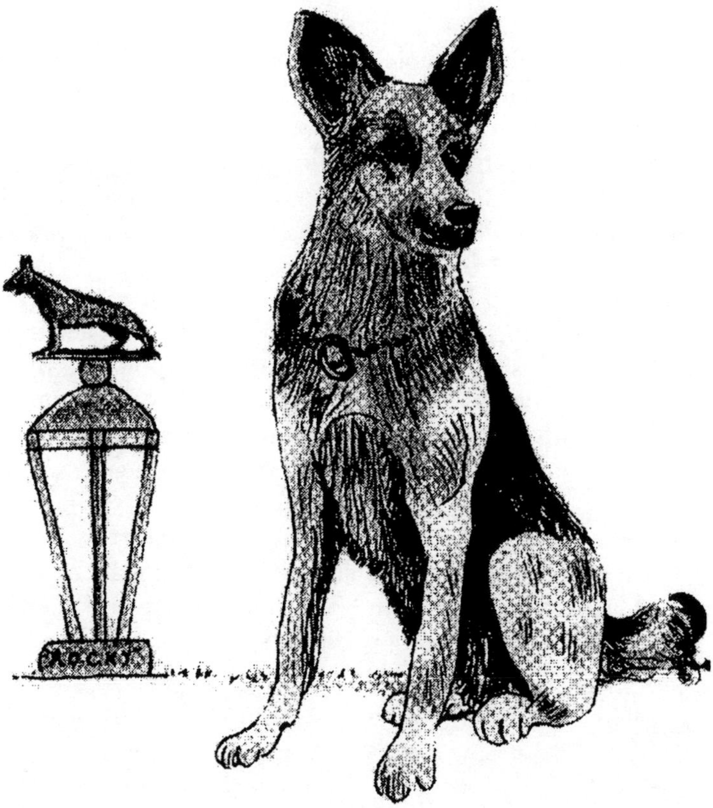

ROCKY AND ME

I bought this pup and brought him up, I trained him for the trials
to be the best to win the cup, for this we traveled miles.
My memories of him never dim, he was more than just a dog,
all my time was spent with him, as mist does with the fog.
Day and night we practiced long, it was a tedious grind.
At first, it all went wrong, I though I'd lose my mind,
'cause Rocky did not understand, he only wished to play.
Even on my reprimand he still would want his way.

Now, this went on for many a day, and then, but not complete,
he would respond to what I'd say, but not without some treat,
but Rocky came to know that treating wasn't all,
my voice came firm but softly low was all I need to call.
Our lasting friendship strongly grew into one solid bond.
Time came soon that we would know that both of us were fond,

of what is just a simple game, an exercise at best;
to win the judge's apt acclaim and pass his drilling test.
To be the best dog in the shows to take the winner's cup,
an acclamation that bestows upon me and my pup.
I taught him all the moves and tricks a happy dog it makes,
for this contentment oft' restricts many of our mistakes.

While training in obedience this fact remained to be:
that doing this experience, same things for him and me,
For wisely smart was Rocky, no smarter dog than he,
'cause while I was teaching Rocky, Rocky was teaching me.
We both were learning self control, him, much better than I.
From out of the past memories unfold, lasting until I die.

He was placed on any beat, a sit, a stand or lie,
not even a bitch in cycle heat could steal a glancing eye!
He would respond to my command, a voice or hand it be,
he'd clear the highest jumping stand and then return to me.
I would touch a special thing of metal, of leather, or wood,
and Rocky knew which one to bring for Rocky understood;

That in that pile of fifteen, placed without inspection,
(cause Rocky had not seen)
he just used his scent detection with nose so sharply keen.
Proudly wagging his tail in glee when snatching up the one,
the only one that's touched by me, and back to me he'd come,

Returning this item back to me, he came in joyful prance -
his eyes as wide as could be, his pupils in a dance!
Since all this happened long ago and Rocky is now gone,
many thoughts I have in stow, I'll never be alone!
Rocky left us while in glory he was just a young pup then...
met his maker, (without gory) upon a road his life did end,

but not before he captured many cups and titles that he won;
hearts of love and praise a plenty, all agree a job well done.
So from the days of yesteryear comes thoughts of Rocky's skill.
All our memories now revere...in all our lifetime fill.

❖❖❖❖❖

GONE BUT NOT FORGOTTEN

Go back in time to my young prime, to 1935,
when I was just a lad of nine; when songs were juke box jive.
No wars or sparks were in our midst; just peace and harmony.
No matter where the folks exist, we all felt good and free.
I lived at 5th and Castle Street where life there grew most fond,
everyday a special treat on sidewalks of "dry pond!"
We played each day and sometimes night without a thought of fear.
With skates or bikes there on the site, few cars were ever near.

We ran or walked to our downtown or rode a city bus,
five cents a trip there all around was quite alright with us.
About that time there chance to be just one good fad around,
long ago before TV, when no drugs could be found.
No smoking pot, no sexy shows, no drive-by shooting sprees;
just shooting marbles with our foes, and doing so with appease.
Now this game was very simple, we bunched 'em in a ring,
burst 'em like a pimple, then watched the marbles spring!

If any marble left the ring, you then continued on...
until you missed or came to bring... a so-called "marble run".
So when you picked up all there was, leaving opponents none;
a "wizard" then you're called because of all your marbles won!
We showed-up with a brilliant scheme, at least that's what we thought;
until appeared upon the scene a lesson we were taught!
Far from the past this tale I cast,
coming from memory lane; an unknown name
whose marble game made all our egos wane.

'Twas on one early summer morn we chose a spot to play,
the best of shooters true to form to win the crown that day.
We played about a half a day, my pockets all filled up;
I believed I'm on my way to win the champion's cup,
but then appeared a little guy without his shoes and socks,
his eyes as blue as summer's sky, had white-hair curly locks.
This boy was barely four feet tall, a new kid on the block;
no problem here I saw at all, I thought he'd go in hock!

But on his face a cocky sneer, just like a red sly fox,
he smartly grinned from ear to ear, and clutched an empty box.
His hands looked like two T-bone steaks that held five marbles there;
for four was all it took for stakes and one for shooting sphere.
His hands showed wear from constant dare, a "tough one" he must be;
for spots of blood shown here and there, came from his hand and knee.
And when he cocked his huge right thumb to let the shooter go,
I realized then his shot to come, would be a mighty blow!

The shot he fired, a trembling blast, caught everybody's eyes...
...for half the marbles rolled out fast, and left us in demise.
Then he commenced to settle down to shoot the others out.
With one knee there upon the ground,... the game became a rout!
I never saw so much grace displayed by anyone,
he moved in such a splendid pace; and made his shooter run;
also made his shooter spin, go left, go right or stop!
all to gain a spot within to win the marble crop.

So in the end he filled his box; and crowned the king was he;
and by the hands of Grandpa's clock comes my strong memory,
and here there was a lesson learned; which you can always bet:
no matter how much skill you've earned; there's someone better yet!!

❖❖❖❖❖

SCHOOL DAYS

Here is a tale of my school days from many years gone by;
recalling some exciting ways when life was at a high.
I will not cite the sometime lows, only the highs recalled,
for I'm too old to dwell on woes and keep from going bald!
But, how I miss those happy years when everything was bright,
folks could walk without their fears, the lonely streets at night.
I would rise in early morn with school class on my mind,
knowing there would be no scorn- just loving friends to find.
I must confess I loved it so for now I will admit;
that many times I left to go to school while darkness sit,

and many times I went before my Mom got out of bed,...
quietly, sneaking out the door before the light was shed.
I had to reach the school yard as early as I could;
not for good marks on my card, but play games that felt good.
There was one game called "Gotta Go", with one side in a ring;
the other side, of course the foe...was there to try and bring...
...the kids who left that marked-out spot to place them at a tree...,
and on a grasp, which they got, would shout one two and three!
And then when caught and put in line, stretched out beneath the tree,
the sides would change 'less came around, a kid to "set 'em free!"

Now, this was done by just a touch to some hand in that line...
and this is why I loved it much, this game of youth divine,
for it was me they usually missed for I was known to be;
the one they chased and came to list; "The kid who set 'em free!"
I was quick and swift as rabbits run...could dodge with skill galore;
no grasp they got because I spun--, and missed me as before.
So memories of my years in school, they linger ever yet...
back living by the golden rule and having no regret.
Just sweet memories of my youth when in the early grades,
the hero of the day, Baby Ruth, was riding in parades.

Later, in my high school years life got better still,
for in those times there were no fears...just happy times to fill.
We all were one big family, how great it was back then...
for what was once a graceful spree, is not a modern trend!
Of high school teammates that I had, I'll only cite just two.
The first, a very super lad, had talent through and through.

Diminutive, demonstrative, but he was not a clown,
he was good in all he did, his name was "Weenie" Brown.
Now "Weenie" was a little guy but strong as he could be.
He only stood just five feet high, a tiny giant was he.
When in his hands, the basket ball, all fans became aroused,
for on the court from net to net "Weenie" was like a mouse!
He could dribble and run with lightning speed, his moves, the best bar none...
forcing foes to stop and heed, to guard him was no fun.

There was one act that he did thrive when chased all o'er the gym...
he would fool the other side with pass to teammate Tim, who suddenly dunked it in!
On baseball's mound, "Weenie" was sound, quite a pitcher was he,
for not too long all batters found, his pitch they could not see!
Of second friend I'm just as fond, no skills were ever truer,
for it was football he did bond...his name was "Homer" Brewer.
Now "Homer" thrilled the multitudes that came to see him treat...
with reckless movements in his runs brought crowds up to their feet,
and "Homer" ran with lighting speed and good at changing pace...
just where he'd go no one could heed...he led them in a race.

While running with a tricky call and at the line was stuck;
he had a way of fooling all by waddling like a duck,
and before the tacklers knew it, his route wound change with dare,
and the puzzled defense would "blow it" for "Homer" would sail on air...
over many would-be tackles...and players left standing there...
no way they're going to shackle for "Homer" is on a tear.
Now you could see a lot of men sprawled out upon the ground...
too late for them to up-end, 'cause "Homer" is touch down bound!
Now it feels so good in looking back to reminisce a while...
for nothing in this world I lack...are memories that I file,
but most of all it feels so great...having gone all through that phase,
is convey to you and celebrate my early youth school days.

❖❖❖❖❖

TODAY'S TREASURES, TOMORROW'S TRASH

"Great day! What a mess up here!"

How many times I used those words I can't venture to guess upon entering the attic, garage, or some other storage area in our home. I can't begin to count the times I've moved storage "junk" from one place to another just to make room for more. Sometimes, and I'm sure it happens to a million other people, I would come across some item or box of items that had escaped my memory for several years.

In this one particular case I describe in my poem, "Today's Treasures, Tomorrow's Trash." We actually hauled and stored that "stuff" for 30 years! I finally focused in on those belongings, or "valuable junk" is probably a better term, and discovered the many items described in the poem, but I guess like the poem indicates, we're stuck with it!

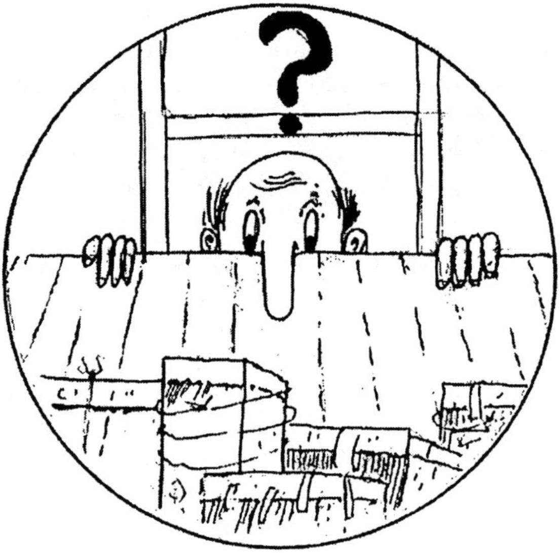

TODAY'S TREASURES, TOMORROW'S TRASH

Should your day become depressing
And you want to change your view,
Go up into your attic and search it through and through,
And you will find your worries decreasing to just few,
By finding some things up there that once were part of you.

When I entered into mine to clean things up for spring,
I came upon some boxes and curiosity it did bring!
I brushed away the cobwebs that to those cartons clung;
Across to near by rafters where other items hung.

My anticipation soared as I opened up a box;
The first things I discovered were our children's baby socks.
Next, their baby clothes and a dehydrated rose,
Also hair from curly locks.

A pack of pacifiers, some Sears & Roebuck "flyers"
And a book by Dr. Spock, the one on chicken pox.
Other little frilly things like underwear with laces;
A coat or two, some dresses blue in two worn out suitcases.

Some pairs of jeans some blues and greens,
And some had stain-like traces.
A game of rook, a photo book
Of babies smiling faces!

Also Baby shoes in bronze, uniforms they'd donned.
They now restore my thoughts of all that we were fond.
Both sons and me in little league as coach and players bond.
I found baseball mitts, some bats and kits, all from me they'd conned!

All our children are now grown, married with their own.
Forgotten were these tokens buried in cardboard's tomb!
These souvenirs bring on the tears which grips me to the bone,
But now I see my wife and me realize a job well done!

Another box, inside some frocks, and gown of long ago,
Recalls my bride in slowly stride, her face in all its glow!
I found her shoes still shinny bright and Bible yet as white,
With orchid dried below its bow, and photos of the site
At reception's champagne flow.

Beneath that stack, my trousers black, a tie and coat of white.
Other clothes I thought disposed and shoes that felt too tight.
A wallet worn and britches torn when bending o'er that night.
All this stuff has lasted tough, lost and long from sight.

Other things discovery brings makes my day complete;
Old picture frames and model trains and set of drums we beat.
Crafts we made now dull and frayed, boxed up head to feet!
My scrap books show that long ago I made my youth complete.

As I look around I'm duty bound to keep these items stored;
"Cause come those days which have dismays I'll keep from being bored,
But in due time someone will climb and move this worthless store--
To some land fill beneath some hill-- beyond our trumpet's roar.

❖❖❖❖❖

A WESTERN DREAM

In September 1988, my wife, Bobbie, and I took a trip by car to San Diego, California to visit our daughter and son-in -law, where he was stationed in the Navy. At first, I was skeptical about traveling that far for a couple of reasons.

One, I was still recuperating from open heart surgery and two, I had a history of vertigo and was leery of high places. The fact that I had never been near a mountain caused me no small concern. I really did not know what to expect. I had always wanted to do this, but the opportunity never presented itself.

So now it did and off we went. I have to say it was the best experience that I've ever known. While I could write volumes about this trip, I'm hoping my short poem, "Western Dream," will significantly tell you about this journey.

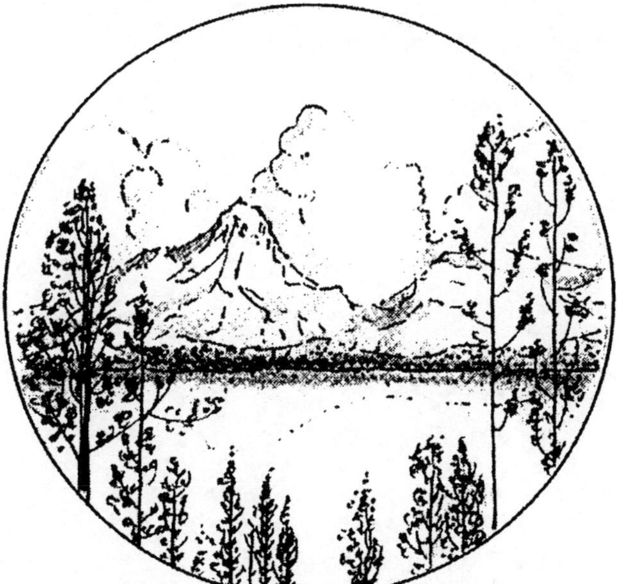

A WESTERN DREAM

I drove across our western land beneath its spacious skies;
around its span of mountains grand where all its wonder lies.
I did not fly by aeroplane, from down I wished to see
the many thinks that nature brings in all their beauty be.
Just like a boy's first trip to town, I'm struck with rapturous awe;
I felt amazed as out I gazed at miracles that I saw.

I saw the mighty mountains rise stretched out across the range.
I viewed the brilliance of their hue beyond the sprawling plains;
and looking there across the plains I felt my freedom rise;
for in my heart a joy will start of scenes that met my eyes.
I felt this joy just like that boy whose ego's on the soar!
I realized a paradise I never saw before.

Carrying on I wasn't alone, I felt that God was nigh
as I rode the brim of rock and rim that peaked along the sky;
and the many wonders of the land I viewed with humble pride;
Death Valley sand to Canyons Grand, out to the Great Divide!
The splendors of the forest greens, the waterfalls in view;
the beauty of the loving things which makes our dreams come true.
These final words you must take heed and note this vital tip:
"Do not fly, but with due speed, you owe yourself this trip!"

❖❖❖❖❖

YESTERYEAR'S INFLATION

First, let me say that I think that everything, and I mean everything in the country that drives and controls our lives is money. The old saying, "Money is the root of all evil," is not true. "Money is the root of all our lives." It's not a matter of rich and poor, because this is only a result of the efforts of these individuals. Everyone just has to do the best they can.

Unfortunately, as we all know, money has been at the root of all evil greedy people. Money is the backbone of our American System, and with the freedom it brings, I wouldn't have it any other way.

However, looking back over the years it simply amazed me how far inflation has brought us. In this simple poem, "Yesteryear Inflation," I merely indicate how the cost of living has had such tremendous surge over the years.

YESTERYEAR'S INFLATION

The cost to live was almost naught in days of way back when,
and I will share some of my thoughts about that time and trend.
It only took a ten cent piece for any show in town,
and while in there a nickel's fare bought popcorn by the pound!
And movie flicks were not as sick as those you see today,
the stars were super like Gary Cooper and beaut's like Alice Faye.

A bus to town, a nickel a round, to shop a ten cents store.
A quarter would buy a silk neck tie, well, who could ask for more?
Not anytime was spent in line when in the grocery stores,
and the clerks were good in bagging food and also opened doors.
The butcher's shop we stopped a lot, no lower price was found,
a pound of chops, 20 cents top..., and fat-back...five cents a pound!

A pepsi ad was soft drink's fad and it certainly hit the spot,
for just a nickel our thirst buds tickled 'cause twelve ounces was a lot!
Just one cent was all one spend for just one cigarette,
and brand new cars was cheap as jars when two thousand all one net.
Well, we've come a long way since my hey day, with cost now out of sight,
and I will say without delay, it will never again be right!

❖❖❖❖❖

BATTLE OF BUBBA AND ME

In 1990, we moved to Belhaven, North Carolina, where we were fortunate enough to buy waterfront property located on the Pungo River. This gave me the opportunity to fish more conveniently, and we always dreamed of just living on the water for beauty's sake. However, perhaps of the location, fishing wasn't all that productive and although I managed to have a lot of fun with the "average" size, I always continued with the hope that the "big one" would come along.

It wasn't until a friend told me of an old gentleman that operated a borrow pit on his 30 acre farm, about 10 miles from my house. He had stocked the excavation with many species of fish after the water had naturally filled in. It was learned later that a hurricane had created a flood in nearby Pamlico Sound causing the overflow onto this man's reservoirs. This overflow not only stocked the pit but brought many species of sea-life as well.

I was elated when I heard of this. Off I went to obtain the gentleman's permission to fish his three lakes! Can you imagine, it was a fisherman's dream come true. When he gave me the okay, I had to pinch myself. The area was a secluded rural section and I pretty much had it all to myself.

The verse, "Battle of Bubba and Me," is described as close as I can get to the actual truth in my catch. Every fisherman, and I'll say without reservation, dreams of catching one like Bubba. It was my dream come true.

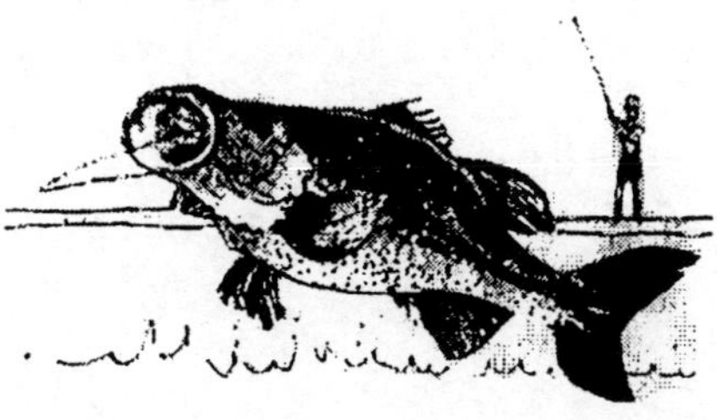

BATTLE OF BUBBA AND ME

I believe there comes a time In everyone's heart and mind,
A strong wish for something fine where some failing is assigned,
But winning out by great divine by keeping one's nose to the grind.
This is the way for me it began. I'll try to tell it the best I can.
I went for a short drive in my van for all the scenery my eyes could scan.
As I drove along that summer morn, my eyes caught sight of this field of corn,
And beside that grain a path was torn through thick of bushes, and weeds it borne.
Curiosity led me down that trail where I was startled by flushing quail.
A feeling came high, my heart did swell, a sense that something will soon unveil.
Upon my arrival filled with hype I was overcome with great delight,
Beyond that field a beautiful sight, a pond of water back there lay quiet.
Only sound came as geese took flight. Wait! I hear something, some splashing sound,
And when I spun to look around, couldn't believe what I just found
a big mouth bass at least ten pounds! He broke the surface of this yawning lake
To capture food within his wake. For one large fish this one takes the cake! In my pounding heart he's mine to take.
I rushed to the van to get some line 'cause I knew this fish would soon be mine,
I will find out that life is not kind for my tackle had been left behind!
I regret, but I won't dismay, 'cause I'll be back another day,
And I shall return as MacArthur did say. I'll come tomorrow in search of my prey.

Well, tomorrow did come, which is today, and anxiously I travel along my way
Back where I saw that big fish play. I can't wait to get there, I must say.
With me I brought a variety of bait. I wanted to be sure to seal his fate.
I brought spinners, twisters, all up-to-date. I laid out my plan to lay in wait.
(I even brought scales to be sure of his weight!)
Now I'm ready to cast out my reel, nothing but good fortune do I feel.

A matter of time his fate will seal. Out went my lure in search for my thrill.
Upon the hook the best worm around, made of plastic, but proven sound.
It wiggles, it squirms, it twists and bounds, until this big mouth gulps it down!
I am tipping my rod hoping by chance Big "Bubba" will see that worm in dance,
Chase the worm bait and on him do prance, and relieve me of my wide-eyes trance!
Several hours pass nothing is sure. I guess it's best for another lure.
I'll go to a spinner, something newer. How can we miss? The water so pure.
Out goes the "Popper" best plug there is. It gurgles, and bubbles, it's a whiz.
This one must be a favorite of his. I really don't want this one to miss.
Now the hour is late the shadows long. There must be something I've done wrong.
I see some small ones all in a throng. It means that "Bubba" may come along.
Suddenly! and with a jerking snare came a tug at my line, nothing to spare!
"I've got 'em now," I react with flair, this tom-tom heartbeat I cannot bear.
He darts and dives and my line does tear!
Just as suddenly as time was spent I felt this terrible pain which lent
to the very fact my line was limp. My sick heartstrings were never so bent,
'cause Big "Bubba" just got up and went!
He got away with a forced display, but tomorrow is another day.
I know exactly where he will stay, and when tomorrow comes he will pay!

Here I stand on the banks of this pond, one which I've built a very strong bond,
Hoping that "Bubba", whom I am fond will take this hook on my fishing wand.
Now "Bubba" is slick and seems to know precisely who are his foes.
He has shunned my spinner I did throw, and to the worms turned up his nose.

A small fish now I hang on my hook to dangle it in front of his nosy snook,
Swimming and darting with natural look so Big "Bubba" refuses to spook.
I stand now gazing across the way enjoying the warm summer's day;
Watching my "Bobber" in its motion's sway, brought by the bait fish in its play.
Then without warning the "Bobber" dived. Suddenly, I knew "Bubba" arrived.
I am not going to be deprived; it's a fight to the finish, dead or alive!
He pulling hard, I dare not reel for fear that "Bubba" may try to steal.
Now I'm thinking hard with all my skill; I want "Bubba" to enjoy his meal.
No "Bobber" seen yet, I have him still.
Now I am reeling with a steady grind. My heart is jumping, I can hardly wind.
Come to me "Bubba", you're mine, you're mine! My dream has come true, The one I opine!
As he approached I could see him clear. He looked the size of a cubby bear.
His scales were black and shiny like hair, and in his mouth small fish...still there!
He was holding on with all his might, and there is no way I could sight.
All I know is there was a fight. One look at me and he took off in fright!
For after he grabbed that little bait fish he did not swallow it for his main dish,
That big sharp fish hook as was my wish. I didn't expect it to end like this!
I just can't explain the emptiness that brought a swelling up in my chest.
I think I'll need to go home and rest, after this, I believe rest is best.
But I am going to get him yet! Within my lifetime I surely bet,
and if it takes all of my sweat, this guy will know his match was met.

Now for the fourth time I'm back again. Three times I lost him and three times pain.
Very evasive this trail he has lain. Today is the day if it doesn't rain.
Now patience is virtue I've been told. Be smarter than others in the fold.
I'm not leaving 'til "Bubba" is cold. He will be riding my cooler behold!

With confidence built and method the same, not making excuses, not showing blame,
Just fishing for "Bubba" who brought me shame. Catching "Bubba" today is mainly my aim.
I've been here now for about an hour. I'm 'bout ready to go home and shower;
'Cause at the top of my golden tower I've been blessed like God's little flower.
Now in my home I stand-up tall where here I suffer no more appall,
For I have answered the mighty call, and above my mantel he does sprawl,
"Bubba", who is mounted on my wall!

JACK OF ALL TRADES

All my life I've been a procrastinator. I'm not proud of that -- in fact, I don't think I knew its real meaning until recent years. I've always involved myself in all sorts of activities as I came along. On everything I set out to do I would try to give it 100 percent. I never really concentrated on any one particular thing. Sports, art, carpentry and music were just a few things that I did well. However, in my later years, I began to regret that I did not expand. In the following poem, "Jack of All Trades," I explain this a little further

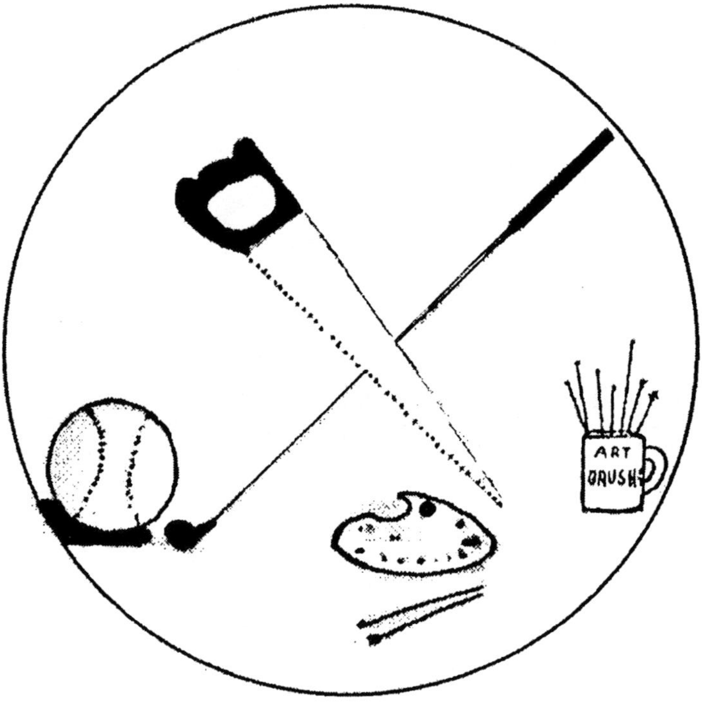

JACK OF ALL TRADES

I'm a Jack of all trades, master of none of many chores of skill,
and when it comes to do just one, I'm strickly "run of the mill".
I'm Jack of all trades, master of none, but best at what I do,
I go all day with run, run, run, and work the whole day through!

I'm a Jack of all trades, master of none, and I've 'bout done it all,
and when it comes to work for fun I surely had a ball!
As Jack of all trades, I'll list a few, but don't expect them great.
I'm just one man, a one-man crew who has much to relate.

When I was eight I was a marble champ great, a wizard in my time,
but, put to the test 'twas laid to rest...dethroned at age of nine.
And as a lad I couldn't be had as ping-pong champion too,
but in short time 'twas just a fad and I did not follow through.

When I was young and in my teens 'twas no one proud as I,
for out I went and made all teams, but I kissed those skills goodbye,
in oils, I've painted a thousand scenes but none have brought a name,
but they have made some folks serene and I will accept the same!

I'm an artist, a painter, and a carpenter too, but never given any parades;
but I had the strength to see it through as a "Jack of all trades".
Golf is the game that I play best, but I never gained my fame,
I could always score as well as the rest, but never received acclaim!

So here I am at the end of my line, there are no regrets say I,
For everything in my life is fine; there's nothing left to try!
Now I've lived my life and filled it up and after all is said and done,
As Jack of all trades I filled my cup although I mastered none!

MACO LIGHTS

About 30 miles southwest of Wilmington, NC there lies a town named Maco, NC. It was there that a strange phenomenon began many years ago. To this day the suspense of that mystery continues.

It is alleged that a brakeman, while on duty one night, lost his life when he accidentally slipped and fell below his train and was beheaded. The legend goes that he returns only on nights with certain conditions to retrieve his head. While this is a gruesome and suspicious tale, it was said that concerned officials investigated it by blocking traffic and shutting lights down in order to solve the mystery. However, to this day it's still not explained. These lights do exist. I've seen them myself, and they can also be attested to by hundreds of other people who claim they too have seen the lights. At any rate, the verse, "Maco Lights," says it all!

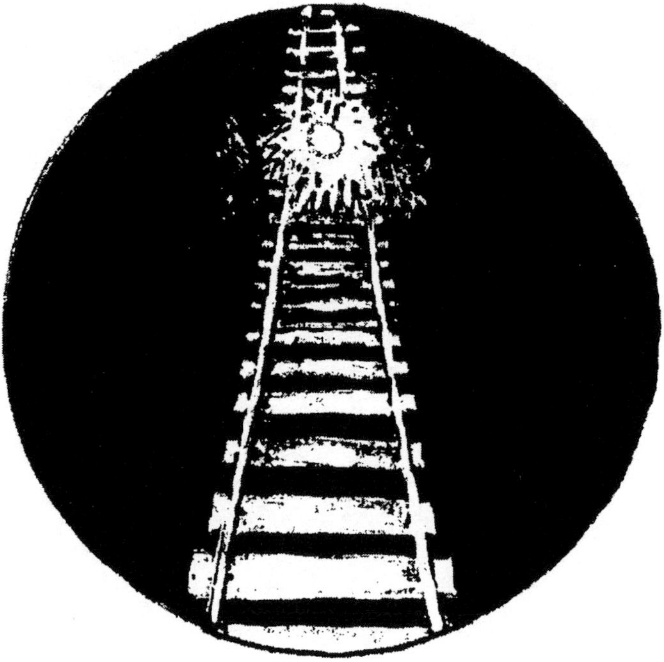

MACO LIGHTS

'Tis said that many years ago in a North Carolina town;
A brakeman slipped and fell below the wheels of a western bound,
And each night near this Maco site, a search goes on, 'tis said,
Of a brakeman's plight by a lantern's light, to find his missing head!

And people come from miles around to see this strange affair.
They come to town with silence bound to view the lantern's glare.
It seems to show the weirdest glow which flickers in and out,
Swinging 'round and to and fro, constantly all about!

A ghostly tale of stretch of rail that chills the strongest spines.
Of those who come, all will fail to know why this light shines.
The night must be as black as tar to view this mystery sight;
For just a wink of one bright star could blind the Maco light.

A cloudy night when you can't sight your hands before your eyes;
Is better chance that time is right -- for lamplight on the ties.
And many experts near and far have tried to solve it out,
By blocking every light and car for many miles about.

Still yet it shines along the lines about the railway bed.
Looking, searching for some signs of that brakeman's missing head!
As the light draws near you can hear the footsteps as they squeak,
Your heartstrings sear as you freeze in fear that you can hardly speak!
Then quickly there right in thin air, silence steals the glows,
It disappears within a stare, and where it goes -- nobody knows!

❖❖❖❖❖